Doctors, Diseases and Opera

Dr J. Ian S. Robertson

Dr J. Ian S. Robertson FRS(Edin.), MD, FRCP(Lond.), FRCP(Glas.), FAHA, FIBiol., BA(Manc.) is a former Professor of Medicine whose particular interests were in cardiology, hypertension, and endocrinology. Following retirement he gained a BA with first-class honours in Opera Studies at the University of Manchester. From 1999 to 2008 he was a member of the board of directors of Scottish Opera. He has written and lectured widely on medical aspects of opera.

First published in 2019 by Nostrebor Publications, 9/1, 205 Albion Street, Glasgow G1 1RU, UK

A CIP record for this book is available from the British Library

ISBN 978-1-5272-3673-8

Front cover: *Pelléas et Mélisande*, Scottish Opera, 2017. Photo: Richard Campbell. Back cover: *Otello* (Verdi), Scottish Opera, 1972. Photo: Bob Anderson.

Typeset in Garamond by Core Image Graphics Department.

Printed and bound in Great Britain by Core Image, 5-6 Tennant Avenue, College Milton South, East Kilbride, Glasgow G74 5NA.

CONTENTS

Part III: Two More Operatic Doctors

Part IV: Doctors Writing About Opera

PREFACE

As I explain in more detail in my introductory chapter, *Doctors, Diseases, and Opera* is a complementary companion volume to my earlier book *Doctors in Opera: An Irreverent Look at Operatic Medicine.* That was an account of doctors appearing as characters on the operatic stage. The present book rather differently deals with the remarkably diverse influence of medical men and women on other aspects of the operatic art. Also considered is the involvement of various diseases in operatic plots and their adverse effects on some composers of opera. Additionally I provide accounts of six operas featuring a doctor which I previously omitted, three of them because they appeared too late for inclusion.

I am grateful for much encouragement and generous practical aid from Alex Reedijk, General Director of Scottish Opera. I thank Jeffrey Sharkey, Principal, and Linda Robertson, Communications Officer, Royal Conservatoire of Scotland; Rachel Hynes, opera singer; my editor Ian Brooke; and my secretary Susan Wilkie. I am also greatly indebted to numerous authors whose writings on and around this topic preceded my efforts; these I have attempted to acknowledge in my concluding chapter.

Any remaining faults are mine.

Author's note: All mentions of *Grove* in chapter endnotes refer to *The New Grove Dictionary of Opera* (4 volumes), edited by Sadie, S., Macmillan, London, 1992.

INTRODUCTION

In 2012 my book *Doctors in Opera: An Irreverent Look at Operatic Medicine* was published.[1] This was, as the subtitle states, a not overly respectful account of doctors as they are portrayed as characters on the operatic stage. The work was gratifyingly well received, and proceeded to a second, much enlarged, edition in 2016.[2] I included an introductory chapter dealing briefly with the influence of medical men and women on other aspects of opera: as librettists, composers, conductors, singers, and so forth. However, it quickly became apparent that these latter roles and circumstances merit more detailed appraisal; this I have attempted in the present book, which can be taken as a complementary companion volume to the earlier *Doctors in Opera*.

Herein I describe and evaluate the remarkably diverse ways in which doctors have contributed to the art of opera other than by appearing as characters on stage. Additionally, I consider the involvement of some diseases in operatic plots as well as their pathological effects on a number of composers. I have also taken the opportunity to include accounts of six operas involving a doctor which I previously omitted. *Anatomy Theater*, *The Exterminating Angel*, and *Semmelweis* had their premieres after publication of the second edition. The three others are *The Moon and Sixpence*, *Street Scene*, and *The Lion's Face*.

A number of aspects with which I am presently concerned have been addressed earlier. Ober[3] published a wittily succinct account of the field. Lock[4] provided a broader review, considering, *inter alia*, the impact of various diseases. Also relevant is the book by Hutcheon and Hutcheon, *Opera: Desire, Disease, Death*.[5] The authors are husband and wife, one a physician, the other a literary theorist. They expressly intended 'to combine medical and cultural history with literary and dramatic analyses' in the hope 'that this "concord" might add ... to the understanding of opera's social and artistic impact'. In pursuit of these laudable, if perhaps nebulous, ends, they examined operas dealing with tuberculosis, syphilis, cholera, and cigarette smoking. They also speculated on what an opera concerning AIDS (acquired immunodeficiency syndrome) might offer. At that time no such opera had yet appeared. I found their book to contain several interesting observations. But it was ill-organised, rambling and repetitive. A quotation may give a flavour of their prose: 'To be made self-conscious about the process of how meanings are given – one of the aims of gay countermythologizing – is one step on the way to being more active, daily, in combating stereotyping, stigmatizing, and discrimination.' Their book was generally well reviewed. Marcus, for example, said it was 'scholarly and provocative'.[6] But it certainly provoked another commentator, Charlton, who thought that it was 'an avalanche of constipated gobbledegook'.[7] This was an observation which discomfited both the authors and the reviewer, the latter because his later repute seemed to him to have derived from this one account rather than from his more extensive scientific output.

I have in this present book taken a very broad definition of a doctor. Inevitably, many herein are lapsed doctors, that is, although possessing a medical qualification, they have found subsequently within opera more congenial, interesting, or profitable activities. However, one returned briefly to medical practice after spending several years at musical composition and another after orchestral conducting. Some embarked on medical studies but never qualified. One laid false claim to a medical degree. As shall be seen, I have embraced them all.

1. Robertson, J. I. S., *Doctors in Opera: An Irreverent Look at Operatic Medicine,* Scottish Opera, Glasgow, 2012.
2. Robertson, J. I. S., *Doctors in Opera: An Irreverent Look at Operatic Medicine*, 2nd enlarged edition, Scottish Opera, Glasgow, 2016.
3. Ober, W. B., 'Operatic *"Doctors"*, *The Practitioner* 1976; 216: 110–16.
4. Lock, S., 'Opera', in *The Oxford Illustrated Companion to Medicine*. Edited by Lock, S., Last, J. M., and Dunea, G., Oxford University Press, Oxford, 2001, 593–4.
5. Hutcheon, L., and Hutcheon, M., *Opera: Desire, Disease, Death*, University of Nebraska Press, Lincoln, USA, 1996.
6. Marcus, A. J., review of *Opera: Desire, Disease, Death, New England Journal of Medicine* 1996; 335: 1163–4.
7. Charlton, B., review of *Opera: Desire, Disease, Death, British Medical Journal* 1996; 313: 1022.

Part 1

DOCTORS AND OPERA

DOCTORS AS AUTHORS

A perhaps surprising, but to me gratifying, circumstance is the number of doctors who have distinguished themselves in literature. Many of their works have then gone on to provide inspiration for composers of opera.

Friedrich von Schiller (1759–1805) was one of the world's great literary figures. The son of a doctor, he qualified himself in 1780. However, he seems soon to have found the practice of medicine uncongenial, and he turned to literature, thereafter pursuing an exalted career as dramatist, poet, aesthetician, and historian. Schiller was not musically inclined, but his writings, especially his plays, clearly inspired composers. At least sixty operas are known to have been based on his works. Examples surviving into the current repertoire are Verdi's *I Masnadieri*, *Luisa Miller*, *Don Carlos*, *La Forza del Destino* and *Giovanna d'Arco*; Donizetti's *Maria Stuarda*; Tchaikovsky's *The Maid of Orléans*; Rossini's *William Tell*; and Puccini's *Turandot*.

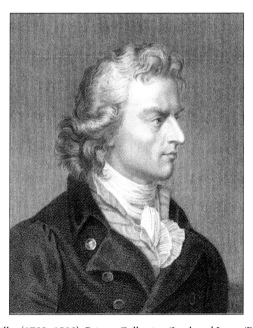

Friedrich von Schiller (1759–1805). Private Collection/Look and Learn/Bridgeman Images.

George Crabbe (1754–1832) was born in the small Suffolk fishing town of Aldeburgh, where his father seems to have combined the duties of customs official, warehouseman, and schoolteacher. Crabbe qualified as a doctor, and for a time practised in Aldeburgh. He seems, however, to have been temperamentally unsuited to medicine, and he abandoned it for the Church, becoming ordained as a clergyman in the Church of England in 1782, concurrently asserting that he had thus transferred to a more ethical and upright profession. That claim I would dispute. The Church did, however, provide him with a secure income and greater leisure time in which he could write the poetry to which he was devoted.

One of Crabbe's poems, *The Borough,* was used by the librettist Montagu Slater for Benjamin Britten's opera *Peter Grimes* of 1945. Interestingly, the two principal characters in the opera, the soprano Ellen Orford and her beloved, the tenor Peter Grimes, are taken from different parts of the original poem, where they never meet. George Crabbe himself is in the opera depicted in a silent role, although other characters address him. In early productions he was called 'Dr Thorp'. The opera is set around 1830 and initially there were worries that having

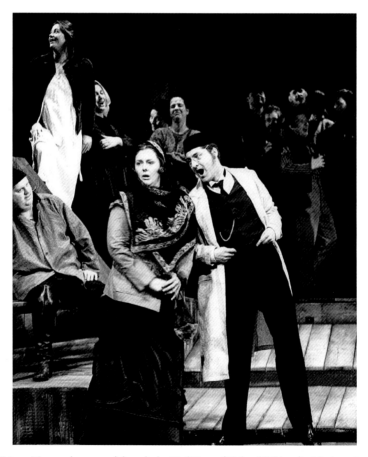

Peter Grimes: The apothecary and drug dealer Ned Keene (Richard Walton) with the opium addict and gossip Mrs Sedley (Catherine Wyn-Rogers). Scottish Opera 1994. Photo: Bill Cooper.

him as 'Dr Crabbe' could be seen as an anachronism. Present-day producers and audiences are less fussy. In the 1830s, unlicensed apothecaries were legally allowed to practice medicine, and in the opera Dr Crabbe has such a rival, the apothecary and opium dealer Ned Keene, sung by a baritone. There are today several memorials to George Crabbe in Aldeburgh. There is Crabbe House, where he is supposed to have lived at one time, and also Crabbe Street.

Georg Büchner (1813–37), whose father and a brother were also physicians, studied medicine at Strasbourg and then at Giessen. By the date of his graduation in 1836, he had already written an inflammatory left-wing revolutionary tract, two plays (*Dantons Tod* and *Leonce und Lena*), a treatise on the nervous system of the barbel fish, and a novella, *Lenz*, concerning Jakob Michael Lenz, who had been a friend of Goethe. Another drama, *Pietro Aretino*, is lost. In 1836 Büchner was appointed lecturer in anatomy in Zürich, but died from typhus shortly afterwards at the age of just twenty-three. After Büchner's death were discovered handwritten fragments of an unpublished play entitled *Woyzeck*, destined to become his most famous work. In 1922 the composer Alban Berg completed the opera *Wozzeck* to his own libretto, which he had prepared from the Franzos edition of Büchner's play. Franzos had originally misread Büchner's almost illegible handwriting; hence the difference between the titles of play and opera. Berg's *Wozzeck*, first performed in 1925, I take to be the finest of all operatic tragedies. Manfred Gurlitt's opera *Wozzeck* appeared just four months after that by Berg. Although initially well received, it has remained overshadowed by Berg's work. Gerhard's *Wozzeck* of 1961 has attracted less attention. Büchner's novella *Lenz* provided the story for the operas *Lenz* by Sitsky and *Jakob Lenz* by

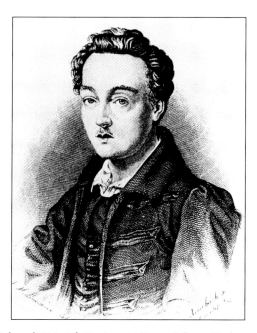

Georg Büchner (1813–37). De Agostini Picture Library/Bridgeman Images.

Rihm. The play *Dantons Tod* was set as an opera by Von Einem. Most favoured with composers of all Büchner's writings is his comedy *Leonce und Lena*. Seven derived compositions are given by Branscombe,[1] although none of these has achieved sustained popularity. Büchner has a lustrous posthumous reputation. Had he survived to maturity he would surely now be ranked alongside Goethe and Schiller among German literary figures.

The Spanish playwright Antonio García Gutiérrez (1813–84) abandoned medicine for poetry and the theatre. Several of his plays were adapted as operatic libretti, most notably his *Simón Bocanegra* of 1843, used by Piave for Verdi's *Simon Boccanegra* of 1857.

Anton Chekhov (1860–1904) continued to practise as a physician throughout his tragically short career. As he famously stated, 'Medicine is my lawful wife and literature is my mistress. When I am tired of one I spend a night with the other.' His literary mistress was remarkably fecund operatically. Chekhov's play *Medved* (*The Bear*) was used in Argento's *The Boor*, Bucci's *The Boor*, and Walton's *The Bear*. His tale *Roman s Kontrabasom* spawned Dubensky's *Romance with Double Bass*, Sauguet's *La Contrabasse*, and Bucchi's *Il Contrabasso*. Another play, *The Proposal*, was the basis of Chailly's *Una Domanda di Matrimonio* of 1957. His short story *Ved'ma* (*The Witch*) is the source of Hoiby's *The Scarf*. Yet another short story, *Rothschild's Violin*, was adapted by Veniamin Fleishman as the libretto for his own opera of the same title, completed by Dmitri Shostakovich in 1944 following Fleishman's death in 1941. Chekhov died from pulmonary tuberculosis, allegedly sipping champagne on his deathbed.

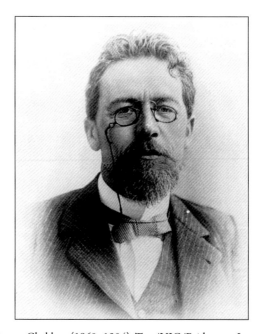

Anton Chekhov (1860–1904). Tass/UIG/Bridgeman Images.

W. Somerset Maugham (1874–1965) wrote a biography of the opera composer Meyerbeer at the age of just sixteen. He graduated in medicine in 1897 but turned aside from that career to be a full-time author of plays, novels, and short stories. Surprisingly little of his considerable output has been taken up by opera composers. There is, however, his novel *The Moon and Sixpence*, set as an opera by John Gardner to a libretto by Patrick Terry in 1957. This opera is discussed later in the chapter on leprosy.

The Ukrainian-born novelist Mikhail Bulgakov (1891–1940) graduated in medicine in 1916 but abandoned that career to pursue writing, wherein he was harshly critical of the Soviet regime. All his publications were banned by Stalin from 1929. Many appeared only years later. His *The Master and Margarita*, an allegorical novel concerning Stalinist repression and terror, was set as operas by Kunad (1986), Holler (1989), and Slominsky (1989). Another satirical novel by Bulgakov, *The Heart of a Dog*, gave rise to operas by Bergsma (1973), Rojan (2007), and Raskatov (2009). The last of these received a lavish English National Opera production in London in 2010.

1. Branscombe, P., *The New Grove Dictionary of Opera* (4 volumes), edited by Sadie, S., Macmillan, London, 1992, I, 629.

3

DOCTORS AS LIBRETTISTS

The preparation of an operatic libretto requires especial skills. A sound basic storyline is an obvious essential. Of necessity, the text is more succinct than that in a corresponding spoken play, yet it must be sufficiently clear to convey the narrative. Most importantly, the verbal structure has to ensure that the musical flow is supported (rather than hindered, which can readily occur) and that dramatic and emotional climaxes are appropriately sited. Crucially, longueurs must be avoided. With all this, the actual words must be appropriate to the singing voice, a vital issue which varies with each type of voice, and most especially with the language being sung. Many operas have foundered on an inept libretto. Weber's *Euryanthe* and *Oberon*, each of which contains some of his finest music, were almost crippled by their inappropriate, inadequate texts. Perhaps surprisingly, doctors have displayed remarkable facility in the preparation of operatic libretti. Grove lists thirteen medical men as librettists, together with two more of rather dubious lineage.[1]

Of these, the Austrian physician Leopold Auenbrugger (1722–1809) deserves particular mention. He graduated at the age of twenty, and proceeded to discover and develop percussion as a diagnostic technique. He had observed that by tapping casks of wine at his father's inn, it was possible, by detecting changes of resonance, to find out how much wine remained. He went on to show that by applying the same method to patients, the outline of the heart could be defined, whether parts of the lung were consolidated by disease, or if there were air or fluid in the pleural space. To minimize discomfort to the patient, when the test is performed the fingers of the left hand are laid firmly on the part to be percussed, usually the chest, and are then struck hard by the fingertips of the right hand. These manoeuvres can often provide an impressive spectacle of medical expertise both to the patient and any watching relatives. In some ways regrettably, the advent of modern imaging methods has now diminished the role of percussion. Auenbrugger's daughter Marianna was a composer and a pupil of Salieri. Auenbrugger himself wrote the libretto for Salieri's 1781 opera *Der*

Rauchfangkehrer (*The Chimney Sweep*). This is a domestic comedy which enjoyed moderate success, albeit Mozart derided the text as 'a miserable piece'.

Two women doctors have each written remarkably skilled operatic libretti. Marie Pappenheim (1882–1966) graduated in Vienna in 1909. In 1909, while still a medical student, she provided the German-language libretto of Schönberg's 30-minute one-act operatic monodrama for soprano, *Erwartung*. The scenario concerns a woman distractedly seeking her lover along a forest path at night. After terrifying experiences, she discovers an object which she fears to be the body of that lover. She calls vainly for help, then expresses fluctuating emotions: sorrow, love, jealousy, tenderness, and compassion. The work ends ambiguously at her words, 'Oh there you are ... I was looking ...'. Of her elusive fantasies Schönberg himself said, 'It is ... the slow representation of things that go through the mind in great anxiety ... the Woman may have been wrong ... there are only fearful imaginings.'[2] Taken with Schönberg's atonal score, which is devoid of formal musical structure, the text conveys vividly the experience of a terrifying dream. It has been widely supposed that Schönberg made substantial emendations to the libretto as composition proceeded. However, Elizabeth Keathley has argued forcibly, if perhaps tendentiously, that Pappenheim's original text remained largely unaltered.[3]

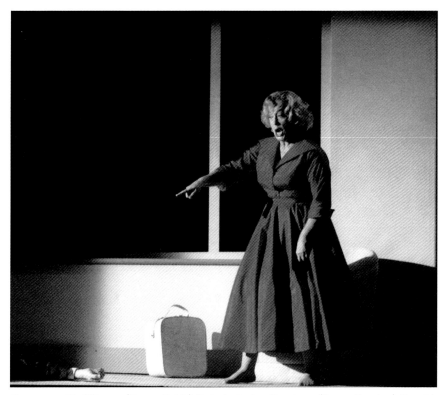

Erwartung: The Woman (Renate Behle) finds the body of her lover (Steven Faughey). Scottish Opera 2004. Photo: Drew Farrell.

Margaret McCartney, currently a working Glasgow general practitioner, wrote the libretto for Gareth Williams' opera *White* of 2009. This is a one-act work, part of Scottish Opera's *Five:15 – Operas Made in Scotland* series. The very brief story is of a foreign hospital cleaner learning English by eavesdropping on a mother comforting her dying daughter. These events, despite their poignancy, are commonplace. Yet the construction of the libretto is supremely accomplished, enabling the composer to convey a vivid musical drama in just 15 minutes.

1. Auenbrugger (1722–1809), Boggio (1738–1816), Castelli (?–1642), David (?–1698), Forzano (1884–1970), Ghislanzoni (1824–93), Jirko (1926–78), Korner (1942–), Moniglia (1624–1700), Neri (?–1726), Ried (1810–69), Salvi (1664–1724), Sardou (1831–1908). Additionally are Frisari (?–1686), referred to several times as 'dottore', and Morselli (?–1691), who has the word 'dottore' handwritten on one title page. *Grove* I–IV, passim.
2. Schönberg, A. Quoted in Cross, C. M., and Berman, R. A. (eds), *Schoenberg and Words: The Modernist Years*, Garland Publishing, New York, 2000, 163.
3. Keathley, E. L., 'Interpreting *Erwartung*: collaborative process and early reception', in Shaw, J., and Auner, J. (eds), *The Cambridge Companion to Schoenberg*, Cambridge University Press, Cambridge, 2010, 81–93.

DOCTORS AS
COMPOSERS

Foremost among composers of opera who have at least dabbled in medicine is Hector Berlioz (1803–69). His father was a doctor who wished his son to follow in that profession. Hector, by contrast, was determined to become a composer of music. Nevertheless, in 1822 he enrolled as a medical student at the Paris Hospice de la Pitié. On his first visit to the anatomy dissecting room '... a

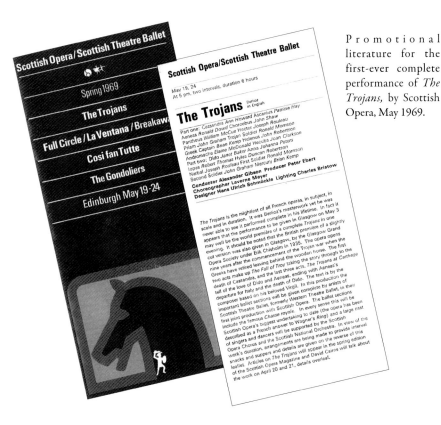

Promotional literature for the first-ever complete performance of *The Trojans,* by Scottish Opera, May 1969.

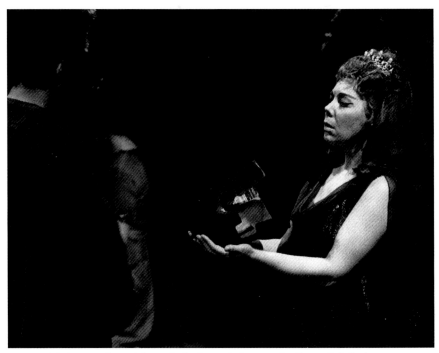

The Trojans: Janet Baker as Dido. Scottish Opera 1969. Photo: Bob Anderson.

feeling of revulsion possessed me ... I did not want to hear another word about anatomy ... or medicine ... I vowed I would be a musician.'[1] And so he became. Sadly his musical genius never in France received in his lifetime the recognition it deserved. What is probably his finest composition, the opera *Les Troyens* to his own libretto, had to wait until May 1969 for its first complete performance, by Scottish Opera in Glasgow. Berlioz is by no means unique as a composer of opera to have abandoned medical studies uncompleted. Many others, albeit less distinguished, are known.[2]

The course taken by Alexander Borodin (1833–87) was very different from that of Berlioz. Borodin graduated in medicine and worked as a surgeon for a year. He then turned to chemistry and was appointed Professor of Chemistry at the St Petersburg Imperial Medical-Surgical Academy in 1864. It was in this field that he was best known in his lifetime and in which he had a most illustrious career. In 1872 he established a medical curriculum for women, a notable achievement in Tsarist Russia. For Borodin, musical composition was a spare-time hobby. Nevertheless, he became a member of Russia's 'Mighty Five' composers, the other four being Balakirev, Cui, Mussorgsky, and Rimsky-Korsakov. During his lifetime few outside that group would have known of his musical talent. Borodin wrote parts of four operas, of which the best known is *Prince Igor*, completed and orchestrated by Rimsky-Korsakov and Glazunov in 1890. Borodin would have been surprised to learn that his posthumous reputation lay in music rather than chemistry.

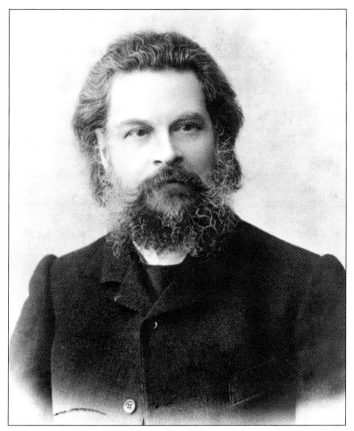

Alexander Borodin (1833–87). Private Collection/Look and Learn/Elgar Collection.

The German-born composer Aquinas Ried (1810–69) is said to have worked as a surgeon at an Australian penal colony for seven years. He then moved to Chile, where, all to his own libretti, he completed four operas plus four others unfinished. All the music is now lost, although the text of one, *Telésfora*, credited as being the first Chilean national opera, does survive.

Leopold Damrosch (1832–85) studied at Berlin University, then abandoned a career in medicine in favour of music. He composed an opera, *Romeo und Julia*, which was performed in Breslau in 1862 but has since disappeared from the repertoire. Leopold Damrosch is now remembered as a conductor rather than composer. He went to New York in 1871 and thereafter played an increasingly important role in the American musical scene. His two sons, Frank (1859–1937) and Walter (1862–1950), both German-born, became naturalized American citizens and notable orchestral conductors.

Bogumil Zepler (1858–1918) likewise deserted medicine after his qualification in favour of musical composition. He wrote a string of operas and operettas, all now virtually forgotten. Zepler was for a time attached to the Berlin Überbrettl cabaret which Ernst von Wolzogen established in 1901, and where many of his songs were evidently popular. Arnold Schönberg was briefly a colleague, and is said to have earned much-needed money by orchestrating some of Zepler's compositions.

The Scottish composer William Wallace (1860–1940) is unusual in returning briefly to medical practice after moving into music. Following qualification as a doctor at Glasgow University, he specialised for a time in ophthalmology – disorders of the eye. He then, in 1889, turned away from medicine to pursue musical composition. He returned briefly to his erstwhile medical speciality during the First World War, then again went back finally and exclusively to music. Wallace is not noted as a composer of opera, although a list of his works includes the one-act lyrical tragedy *Brassolis* of 1896. Wallace's prose writings include the biographical *Richard Wagner as He Lived* (1925) and *Liszt, Wagner and the Princess* (1927), the latter an account of the often fraught inter-relationships between the two composers and Princess Carolyne Sayn-Wittgenstein. Wallace's Irish namesake, William Vincent Wallace (1812–65), who was not medical, is perceived as a composer of operas.

The Ukrainian-born Witold Maliszewski (1873–1939) graduated in medicine at St Petersburg in 1897. He then turned to study music at the conservatory there. He proceeded to teach music, first at the conservatory in Odessa, which he founded, and then as director of the Chopin School in Warsaw. Maliszewski composed two four-act opera-ballets: *The Mermaid* of 1928 to a libretto by Rogowski after a Hans Andersen fairy tale; and *Boruta* of 1930 to a libretto by Oppman.

The Czech composer Ivan Jirko (1926–78) studied medicine and music concurrently at Prague University. He went on to practise as a psychiatrist from 1951 to 1977. He composed four operas, all to his own libretto: *Twelfth Night* of 1964 after Shakespeare; *The Wonderful Adventure of Arthur Rowe* of 1969 based on Graham Greene's *The Ministry of Fear*; and two one-act chamber operas *The Strumpet* and *The Millionairess* of 1970 derived from work of the neorealistic Italian screenwriter Cesare Zavattini.

Giuseppe Sinopoli (1946–2001) was born in Venice and studied music at the Venice Conservatory and at Darmstadt, where one of his teachers was Karlheinz Stockhausen. He also obtained a degree in medicine from the University of Padua and completed a dissertation on criminal anthropology. Sinopoli turned increasingly to musical composition, notably of serial works, and was appointed Professor of Contemporary and Electronic Music at the Venice Conservatory in 1972. His most celebrated composition is the opera *Lou Salomé,* first performed in Munich in 1981. This work, to a libretto by Karl Dietrich Gräwe, tells of the Russian-born Louise von Salomé, psychoanalyst and author, and associate of Nietzsche, Rilke, and Freud. Sinopoli became perhaps even better known as a conductor. He died of a heart attack in April 2001 while conducting a performance of Verdi's *Aida* at the Deutsche Oper in Berlin.

Finally there is the strange case of the Irish composer Joseph Augustine Wade (c. 1801–45), who wrote the very successful opera *The Two Houses of Grenada* of 1826 to his own libretto. Although he claimed to have studied medicine in Dublin, no record of his name appears either at Trinity College or the Irish College of Surgeons.[3] He died young of alcoholism and opium addiction.

1.   Cairns, D. (ed. and trans.), *The Memoirs of Berlioz*, Gollancz, London, 1969, 53–6.
2.   Barbieri (1823–94), Cuyás y Borés (1816–39), Genée (1823–95), Gunsbourg (1859–1955), Kanne (1778–1833), Macchi (1928–92), Martinez (1887–1946), Pierson (1815–73), Schack (1758–1826), Staempfli (1908–2002), von Suppé (1819–95), *Grove* I–IV, passim.
3.   Burton, N., *Grove* IV, 1051–2.

DOCTORS AS CONDUCTORS

Two notable conductors of music, and especially of opera, Leopold Damrosch and Giuseppe Sinopoli, each also composed an opera and are discussed separately in Chapter 4. Zubin Mehta (born 1936) gave up medical study to pursue conducting.

Boyd Neel (1905–81) was born in London and graduated in medicine in 1930. While practising medicine he began musical studies, and went on to form his own orchestra in 1933. This latter venture was successful, and he quitted medicine to devote himself full-time to music. In March 1934 he directed the Boyd Neel String Orchestra, with additional wind players, at the very first operas to be put

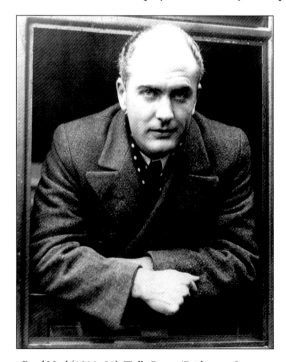

Boyd Neel (1905–81). Tully Potter/Bridgeman Images.

on at John Christie's newly constructed opera house at Glyndebourne.[1] The Intimate Opera Company there performed Bach's *Coffee Cantata* in the operatic adaptation known as *Love in a Coffee Cup*; Mozart's *Bastien und Bastienne*; and Pergolesi's *La Serva Padrona*. Boyd Neel returned briefly to medical practice during the Second World War, thereafter resuming his musical career, mainly as a conductor, then latterly as an administrator.

Jeffrey Tate (1943–2017) was born in Salisbury. He graduated in medicine in 1964, and embarked on a career in ophthalmology. He then abandoned medicine and became a singing coach and répétiteur at the Royal Opera House, Covent Garden. His talents at conducting, especially of opera, blossomed. His international conducting debut was at the Metropolitan Opera, New York, in 1979. He was appointed principal conductor at the Royal Opera House in 1986, and was then their principal guest conductor from 1991 to 1994. From 2005 to 2010 he was music director of the San Carlo Theatre, Naples. Tate was born with the spinal deformity spina bifida. He was also homosexual. The gay scene traditionally reveres physical beauty; hence he saw himself as doubly handicapped. If so, these were impediments he overcame superbly. He came to rank among the finest of contemporary conductors of opera.

---

1.   Hughes, S., *Glyndebourne*, Methuen, London, 1965, 47.

6

DOCTORS AS SINGERS

A surprising number of medical men (they are all men) have taken up operatic singing. I have to concede, however, that the first of these that I shall discuss has very slender credentials for inclusion in a book on operatic doctors.

Theobald Hilarius Marchand (1741–1800) was a German born in Strasbourg. Aged seventeen, he went to Paris to study medicine but then quickly became enamoured of Parisian *opéras comiques* and became instead a singer and actor. He joined a touring company, going on to become its manager. By 1771 their repertoire comprised mostly French light operas in German translation, performed over a touring circuit of Mainz, Strasbourg, Mannheim, and Frankfurt. Marchand nominally retired in 1793 but continued in occasional minor parts until shortly before his death.

Alfred von Bary, of German parentage, was born a British citizen at Valletta, Malta, in 1873. At his father's death in 1877 the family returned to Munich, where the young Alfred studied medicine, graduating in 1898. While working as a junior doctor he began singing lessons, and was found to have a very fine powerful tenor voice. He was persuaded to take up singing as a career and joined the Dresden Court Opera. From 1904 to 1914 he also sang every year at the Bayreuth Festival, performing the major Wagner heldentenor roles to great acclaim. He was reckoned by many to be the finest exponent of Lohengrin to have been heard. He then unfortunately developed severe visual impairment. It has been alleged, albeit as far as I am aware never substantiated, that he had to be guided about the stage by thick inscribed chalk marks. This seems improbable, as he would surely be required to follow the conductor's directions. Von Bary was compelled by near blindness to retire from opera in 1918. He did apparently return briefly to medicine, a circumstance conjuring up the piquant image of a patient startled by confrontation with a doctor who could hardly see him. Von Bary sensibly soon turned aside to seek solace in Catholic theology. He died in 1926.

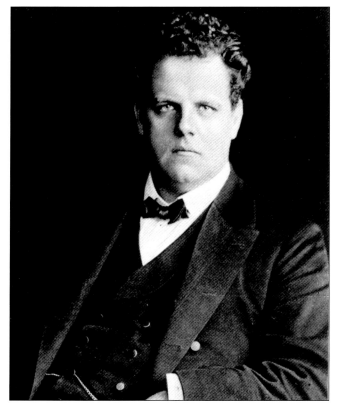

Alfred von Bary (1873–1926). Lebrecht Music Arts/Bridgeman Images.

Richard Mayr (1877–1935) studied medicine in Vienna. He was then persuaded by Gustav Mahler to become a singer. Mayr made his operatic début in 1902 at Bayreuth as the bass Hagen. He was swiftly engaged by Mahler for the Vienna Opera, where he performed for more than thirty successive years. He also had a distinguished international career. Mayr sang the role of Barak in the première of Strauss's *Die Frau ohne Schatten* in 1919 and was a particularly notable Baron Ochs.

The baritone Jules Bledsoe (1898–1943) was born at Waco, Texas. He studied medicine at Columbia University from 1920 to 1924, concurrently having musical tuition. He then abandoned medicine to become a singer, making his professional début in New York in 1924. He created the role of Joe in Jerome Kern's *Showboat* in 1927 and repeated that part in the first film version of 1929. Bledsoe was multilingual and had an impressive vocal range. His operatic career was distinguished, notable roles including Amonasro in Verdi's *Aida*, and the title part in Mussorgsky's *Boris Godunov*. Bledsoe was at different times said to be negro, coloured, black, and Afro-American, although his skin pigmentation remained virtually unchanged. He was one of the first persons answering to those descriptions to sing in opera in the USA.

Vasile Moldoveanu is a tenor born in Romania in 1935. He began medical studies but then turned to singing. Between 1966 and 1971 he performed at the Romanian Opera in roles including Rodolfo (Puccini's *La Bohème*), The Duke (*Rigoletto*), and Tamino (*The Magic Flute*). In 1972 he left Romania and pursued a major international career embracing the Vienna State Opera, Bavarian State Opera, the Metropolitan Opera New York, and the Royal Opera House, Covent Garden. The communist authorities initially considered his leaving the country to be traitorous and he was *in absentia* sentenced to death. There followed rigid censorship in Romania concerning his activities when he was at the height of his vocal career. Consequently, Moldoveanu remains little known in Romania. The political climate subsequently changed. In 2010 his alleged crimes were absolved fully and in 2012 he was made Commander of the Order of the Star of Romania.

The Danish bass Aage Haugeland (1944–2000) studied medicine and music at university in Copenhagen. Music prevailed, and he became a distinguished international singer. His roles included Wagner's Fasolt, Hunding, Hagen, King Marke, and Klingsor; the title part in Mussorgsky's *Boris Godunov*; Ochs in *Der Rosenkavalier*; and the Doktor in Berg's *Wozzeck*.

The contemporary James Gilchrist was a boy treble in the Choir of New College, Oxford, and later a choral scholar in the choir of King's College, Cambridge. He trained, and for a time practised, as a doctor. He turned to a full-time singing career in 1996. Gilchrist is seen principally as a tenor specialising in recital and oratorio singing. Nevertheless, he has performed opera with distinction, notably the title role in Britten's *Albert Herring*.

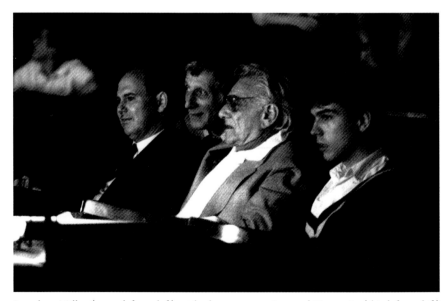

Jonathan Miller (second from left) with the composer Leonard Bernstein (third from left) directing the 1988 Scottish Opera production of *Candide*. Also present are Richard Mantle (first left), general manager of Scottish Opera, and staff conductor Justin Brown. Photo: Eric Thorburn.

7

DOCTORS
AS DIRECTORS

Johannes Schaaf was born at Stuttgart in 1933. He initially studied medicine at Tübingen and Berlin, before turning aside to join the Stuttgart Staatstheater as actor and stage director. During the 1960s he directed also for film and television. He came to prominence in opera with his staging of Richard Strauss's *Capriccio* at the Salzburg Festival in 1985. He then went on to produce a string of Mozart operas at the Royal Opera House, Covent Garden. There followed numerous notable opera productions worldwide. Schaaf's operatic work is described as perceptive, idiosyncratic, and controversial.

Jonathan Miller was born in London in 1934 and graduated in medicine at Cambridge University in 1959. While at Cambridge he was a leading figure in the Cambridge Footlights Revue. In 1960, when still working as a doctor, he helped to write and produce the musical revue *Beyond the Fringe* for the Edinburgh Festival. This launched his major theatrical career. Thereafter Miller became increasingly involved in theatre and television. He began directing operas in the 1970s and went on to become one of the world's leading opera directors with several classic productions to his name. Most striking probably are his 1982 English National Opera Mafia-style *Rigoletto* set in 1950s New York and his 1988 *Candide* for Scottish Opera.

DOCTORS AS IMPRESARIOS AND MANAGERS

The Parisian Louis-Désiré Véron (1798–1867) was a man of considerable business acumen. He made his early fortune as a purveyor of patent medicines, most notably a paste which, when applied to the chest, was purported to cure the common cold. As that malady is self-limiting, the therapy, like many another, was widely perceived as successful. At that time Véron was often referred to as 'Dr Véron', although almost certainly he possessed no medical qualification.

In 1831 the French government decided to relinquish control of the state-controlled Paris Opéra. Véron grasped the financial possibilities. He applied for, and obtained, the franchise, which came with a modest state subsidy. He then brought the talents of designers such as Duponchel; composers such as Meyerbeer, Auber, and Fromental Halévy; librettists such as Scribe and Delavigne; and singers such as Adolphe Nourrit and Cornélie Falcon to create the spectacular genre of Grand Opera. The first new production under Véron's management was Meyerbeer's *Robert le Diable* in 1831, which became an enormous success. When in 1835 the government decided to reduce its financial subsidy, Véron prudently withdrew, having made substantial profits.

Thomas Joseph Walsh (1911–88) graduated in medicine in Dublin in 1944, and became an anaesthetist in the Irish coastal town of Wexford. In 1951, while still a working doctor, he founded the annual Wexford Opera Festival. As nominal artistic director he had a policy of giving the public 'not what it knew and liked but what it might come to like'. There was established a tradition of three works each year: 'one for the head, one for the heart, and one for a little bit of fun'. Initially Walsh personally undertook the selection and engagement of the

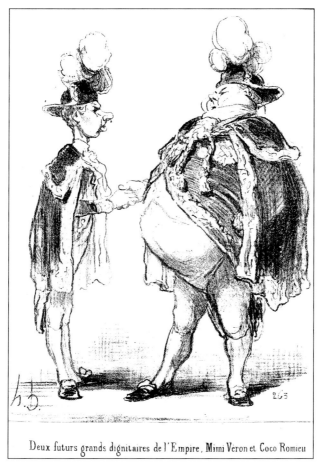

Deux futurs grands dignitaires de l'Empire, Mimi Veron et Coco Romieu

Louis-Désiré Véron (1798–1867) (left) with the French administrator Auguste Romieu, as caricatured by Honoré Daumier in 1851. The caption, with extravagant obsequiousness, describes Véron as 'physician and patron of the arts and letters'. Granger/Bridgeman Images.

principal singers and the training of the local amateur chorus. He retired from the Festival after the 1966 season. Thereafter the directorship became a professional post. The Wexford Festival thrived to become a major annual operatic event. In 2005 a new opera house with enhanced facilities was built on the site of the original theatre. Walsh was also the author of six books on the history of opera variously in Dublin, Monte Carlo and Paris.

The operatic managerial career of Theobald Hilarius Marchand is described in Chapter 6.

Part 2

DISEASES AND OPERA

9

SYPHILIS

To speak of venereal disease in opera almost invariably implies that the disease in question is syphilis. That malady, hugely prevalent worldwide until the late 1940s, was then substantially, but not entirely, eliminated with the advent of treatment with the antibiotic penicillin. Syphilis is caused by the bacterial spirochaete *Treponema pallidum* which is transmitted usually by sexual intercourse. The initial lesion is a hard ulcer, a chancre, appearing on the genitalia within a few days then clearing spontaneously. Some weeks later there erupts the secondary stage involving dispersed inflammation, often ulcerating and painful, in skin and mucous membranes. This too may clear, only to be succeeded after weeks, months or even years by a tertiary phase. In this can appear widespread chronic inflammatory lesions termed gummata. A gumma can affect bone, causing intense chronic pain, or it may ulcerate, with consequent bleeding. There may be cardiovascular disorders, notably incompetence of the aortic valve of the heart. Tertiary syphilis ('the great mimic') can also simulate virtually any neurological disease. In my early medical days in the 1940s and 1950s serological testing for syphilis was mandatory in any patient presenting with a neurological abnormality in which an alternative diagnosis was not immediately evident. Terminally, syphilitic patients often exhibit widespread neurological deficits plus insanity – 'general paralysis of the insane (GPI)'. An interesting feature of syphilis, frequently emphasized in operatic depictions, is that an infecting female carrier may show little abnormality.

SYPHILIS IN OPERA

Richard Wagner's *Parsifal* of 1882 was to the composer's own text. It can be taken that the stricken baritone Amfortas is suffering from syphilis, although this is not explicitly stated in the libretto. Following a sexual exploit with the harlot Kundry (soprano) he has developed a chronic bleeding ulcer in his side and suffers intense bone pain, worsening at night. Both could well result from a gumma affecting a rib and ulcerating through the skin. It must be conceded that

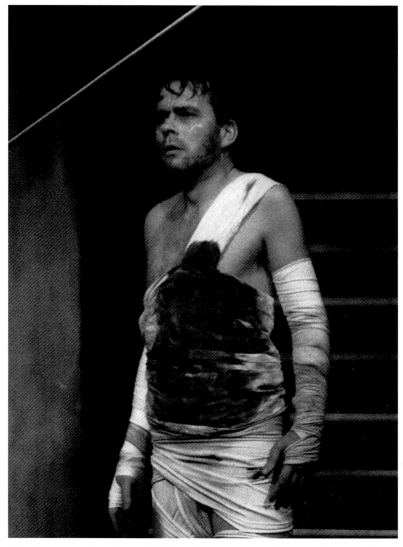

Parsifal: the tormented Amfortas (Matthew Best) with his chronic bleeding syphilitic ulcer Scottish Opera 2000. Photo: Bill Cooper.

at the same encounter with Kundry, Klingsor (bass),[1] the adversary of Amfortas, stole from him the spear sacred to the Knights of the Grail, and then stabbed him with the spear. According to the libretto, that wounding led to the chronic ulcer. Wagner, however, was writing an operatic text, not a medical treatise. In the opera, Amfortas has to wait a very long time for treatment, a circumstance uncomfortably reminiscent of British National Health Service waiting lists. But eventually the tenor Parsifal, who has retrieved the stolen spear, finds his way back, and heals the wound by touching Amfortas with the spear. This might fancifully be seen as a symbolic injection of penicillin. However, Wagner's opera dates from many years before that drug was discovered.

Alban Berg composed the opera *Lulu* to his own German-language text, which he had derived from two plays, *Erdgeist* and *Die Büchse der Pandora* by Wedekind. At Berg's death in 1935 he had completed the entire work in short score, and had orchestrated Acts I and II plus part of Act III. Full orchestration of Act III was eventually achieved by Friedrich Cerha in 1974. The promiscuous Lulu, sung by a soprano, is an evidently symptomless carrier of syphilis. She transmits the disease to the composer Alwa, a tenor. As Alwa states, 'What she caught ... she passed on to me, but she is immune to all the usual symptoms ... who other than she cast me on a bed of sickness and torment?'

Stravinsky's *The Rake's Progress* of 1951 is to a libretto by Auden and Kallman. The dissolute tenor Tom Rakewell engages the services of the Devil, here a baritone going by the name Nick Shadow, for 'a year and a day'. Nick ensures that Tom is infected with syphilis, becomes insane, and is consigned to Bedlam.

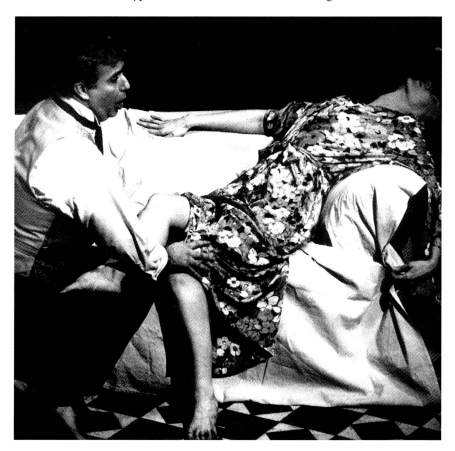

Lulu: The symptomless carrier Lulu (Beverly Morgan) infects Alwa (Eduardo Alvares) with syphilis. Scottish Opera 1987. Photo: Eric Thorburn.

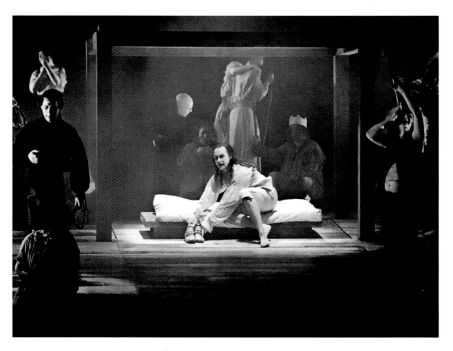

The Rake's Progress: Tom Rakewell (Edgardo Montvidas), insane from tertiary syphilis, is consigned to Bedlam. Scottish Opera 2012. Photo: Mark Hamilton.

The English-language libretto of Leonard Bernstein's *Candide*, derived from Voltaire's French satire *Candide, ou l'Optimisme* of 1762, underwent many major alterations from its unsuccessful New York première in 1956 to the acclaimed Scottish Opera production of 1988. Candide (tenor), a young man living a sheltered life, is indoctrinated with Leibnizian optimism by the philosopher Pangloss (baritone), whose mantra is 'All is for the best in the best of all possible worlds.' Other characters include the maid Paquette (mezzo-soprano), Cunegonde (soprano), and Cunegonde's brother Maximilian (baritone). Pangloss acquires syphilis from Paquette. Pangloss becomes 'an old man with a tin nose ... syphilis has rotted away several of his fingers and left him cruelly disfigured'. Yet Pangloss remains defiantly optimistic:

> Dear boy, you will not hear me speak
> With sorrow or with rancour
> Of what has shrivelled up my cheek
> And blasted it with canker;
> 'Twas love, great love, that did the deed,
> Through Nature's gentle laws,
> And how should ill effects proceed
> From so divine a cause?

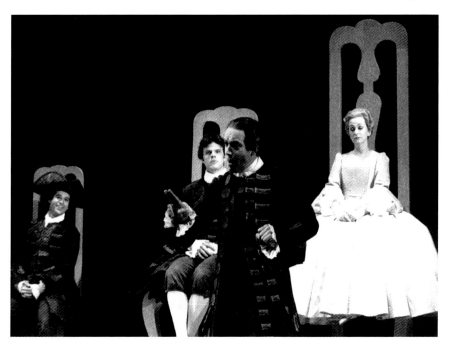

Candide: The syphilitic Pangloss (Nickolas Grace) with (seated, left to right) Candide (Mark Beudert), Maximilian (Mark Tinkler) and Cunegonde (Marilyn Hill Smith). Scottish Opera 1988. Photo: Eric Thorburn.

Giacomo Manzoni's *Doktor Faustus* of 1989, to his own libretto, is based on Thomas Mann's 1947 novel of the same title. Adrian Leverkühn (bass-baritone) becomes a composer of genius by concluding a pact with the devil Him (who constantly changes shape and hence employs a trinity of voices: bass, light tenor and soprano). The price exacted by Him is to have Leverkühn infected with syphilis via the prostitute Hetaera Esmeralda (soprano) and eventually to become insane. In Mann's novel Leverkühn is supposed to have devised the dodecaphonic serial method of composition, which in reality had originated with Arnold Schönberg. Schönberg's angry reaction to the liberties taken by Mann are discussed on page 36. In his opera, Manzoni incorporated the letters of the name of the infecting source, Hetaera Esmeralda, into a note-row which he then deployed via serial composition, reflecting the methodology of Leverkühn and thence Schönberg. Schönberg had died in 1951, however, and was thus spared having personally to endure that indignity.

SYPHILIS IN COMPOSERS

The prevalence of syphilis in the nineteenth and early twentieth centuries was such that it is hardly surprising that it afflicted, or on good evidence was perceived to have afflicted, several prominent composers.

Gaetano Donizetti (1797–1848) was, along with his contemporaries Rossini and Bellini, a leading figure of Italian bel canto opera. Over his career Donizetti composed nearly seventy operas, several of which survive prominently in the present-day repertoire. In 1843 he began to exhibit strange behaviour, with periods of intense nervous excitement alternating with apathy and with inexplicable lapses of memory. He managed to complete *Caterina Cornaro* for the San Carlo theatre in Naples. Thereafter his mental state clearly worsened. His last piece of work was to supply a new ending for the opera for a production in Parma in February 1845. By the autumn of 1845 he was clearly deranged, and was admitted to a sanatorium with a diagnosis of cerebrospinal syphilis. A few months later he had become paralysed and spoke only rarely and then usually disjointedly. He died in 1848. The diagnosis of syphilis was stated to have been confirmed at autopsy.

In 1828 Donizetti had married Virginia Vasselli. She gave birth to three children, none of whom survived. She herself died in 1837 from what has been speculatively described as a 'severe syphilitic infection'.

Despite his brief life, the Viennese late-classical composer Franz Schubert (1797–1828) left a vast compositional oeuvre. It has rightly been said that he ranks among the very greatest of composers in all forms except opera (he wrote no concerti). Of his five operas only one, *Fierrabras*, of no great distinction, receives an occasional performance. In 1823 Schubert developed symptoms of secondary syphilis and began treatment with mercury, then a recognised therapy for the disease. By the mid-1820s his health was however clearly failing; he himself perceived that he was approaching death. By November 1825 he was experiencing headaches, fever, swollen joints, and vomiting. He died on 18 November from what was almost certainly syphilis, although some of his symptoms may have resulted from mercurial poisoning.

The Bohemian Bedrich Smetana (1824–84) is widely regarded as the founder of Czech music. He was predominantly, but by no means exclusively, a composer of operas, of which he wrote eight, with a further one unfinished at his death. At least five of these (*The Brandenburgers in Bohemia*, *The Bartered Bride*, *Dalibor*, *Libuse*, and *The Two Widows*) remain in the present-day repertoire. In 1873 Smetana began to experience steadily worsening symptoms of what was later diagnosed as syphilis. A high-pitched whistling note in his head he apparently introduced into the finale of his E minor string quartet of 1876. By 1874 Smetana had become totally deaf. Although he continued to compose, his symptoms multiplied and worsened. In 1883 he was experiencing varying depression, hallucinations, insomnia, dementia, and dizziness, plus episodes of speech loss. By February 1884 he had ceased to be coherent and was occasionally violent. He was admitted to a Prague lunatic asylum, where he died in May 1884. An autopsy report confirmed the clinical diagnosis of syphilis.

The German composer and critic Robert Schumann (1810–56) wrote just one opera, *Genoveva*. In 1833 he began to experience mental disturbance characterized by depression alternating with elation, plus delusions of poisoning. By 1854 he was having variously demonic and angelic visions. He became aggressive towards his wife Clara. He unsuccessfully attempted suicide by throwing himself into the Rhine and he was admitted to an asylum for the insane. There his mental deterioration steadily worsened until his death in July 1856. Schumann's illness is thought probably to have been syphilis contracted during his student days and remaining latent for a number of years. Poisoning from therapeutic mercury may have worsened his symptoms.

Hugo Wolf (1860–1903), an Austrian composer of Slovene origin is, with Franz Schubert, one of the two greatest composers of German Lieder. His one completed opera, *Der Corregidor*, receives regular, if infrequent, performances. Another opera, *Manuel Venegas*, remains unfinished. A youthful syphilitic infection led in 1897 to insanity. Wolf was admitted to an asylum, where he died in 1903.

Frederick Delius (1862–1934) was an English-born composer of Dutch and German descent. His considerable compositional output includes five operas, four of which, *The Magic Fountain, Koanga, A Village Romeo and Juliet,* and *Fennimore and Gerda*, are occasionally staged. Delius evidently contracted syphilis in his youth. In 1922 he developed the first signs of resultant paralysis. This rapidly progressed, and by 1926 he was blind and physically virtually helpless. He was enabled to continue composing, however, through the assistance of a young musician, Eric Fenby, who volunteered to be his amanuensis.

A COMPOSER WHO PROBABLY DID NOT HAVE SYPHILIS

Wolfgang Amadeus Mozart (1756–91) composed twenty operas plus two uncompleted. Of these, there are six (*Idomeneo, Die Entführung aus dem Serail, Le Nozze di Figaro, Don Giovanni, Così fan Tutte* and *Die Zauberflöte*) which surely rank among the finest ever written. The cause of Mozart's death at an early age has engendered much speculation, most of it wild. In a survey of the literature, Karhausen identified 140 (sometimes overlapping) suggested possible causes of death, in addition to eighty-five other conditions.[2] Syphilis was mentioned only twice, and must be reckoned as a rank outsider. Karhausen also found twenty-seven psychiatric disorders attributed to Mozart. Most of these came from disregarding or mistaking criteria demarcating abnormal from normal behaviour. He concluded that if there were ever a musician who was mentally healthy it was beyond a shadow of a doubt Mozart, in the probable company of Joseph Haydn.

TWO OTHER COMPOSERS WHO DID NOT HAVE SYPHILIS

The Austrian-born Arnold Schönberg (1874–1951) composed in the course of his prolific career four operas, two of which, *Erwartung* and *Moses und Aron*, are regularly performed. He famously devised and introduced the twelve-note serial method of composition. Schönberg's personal qualities included artistic integrity, habitual, but not invariable honesty, and psychological fortitude. Less attractive were egocentricity, belligerence, censoriousness, and suspiciousness, which could readily progress to paranoia. Those latter characteristics were, with some reason, prominently displayed in his breach with the German writer Thomas Mann concerning Mann's novel *Doktor Faustus* of 1947. The central character in the book is a composer, Adrian Leverkühn, who makes a pact with the Devil, becomes a brilliant composer, and devises the dodecaphonic serial method. The Devil's price is to ensure that Leverkühn is infected with syphilis, which then drives him insane. Schönberg was outraged.[3] He had conceived and pioneered that compositional technique, he had never suffered from syphilis, and he was not insane. Schönberg was further angered to learn that Mann's musical adviser had been Theodor Adorno, whom Schönberg disliked and mistrusted. Schönberg died in 1951. He would have been even more upset if he had lived to see Manzoni's opera *Doktor Faustus* of 1989, which was based on, and closely followed, the novel. In that opera, which is discussed on page 33, the serial method of composition is employed by Manzoni.

In later editions of his novel, Mann inserted the grudging acknowledgement: 'It does not seem superfluous to inform the reader that the method of composition ... known as the twelve-tone or row technique, is in truth the intellectual property of a contemporary composer and theoretician, Arnold Schönberg.' Concerning syphilis, Mann was silent.

The extensive oeuvre of Benjamin Britten (1913–76) includes thirteen operas and three church parables, all of which receive regular performances. Britten had a diseased aortic valve of the heart, and in 1973 underwent surgery to replace that abnormal valve. He did not do well. He sustained a stroke at operation, and the replacement valve leaked progressively. He died in 1976.

In 2013 Kildea published a biography of Britten in which he sensationally asserted that at that 1973 operation when the chest was opened the surgeon was surprised to discover that 'the aorta was riddled with tertiary syphilis'.[4] It soon transpired that Kildea's lurid claim was based on the merest hearsay and was wholly untrue. Dr Michael Petch, a cardiologist who had the care of Britten, published a detailed refutation.[5] There was no evidence of syphilis at operation or on histological examination of the diseased valve. Repeated serological tests for syphilis were negative. But no doubt the scurrilous rumour will persist.

1. Klingsor had earlier castrated himself by performing bilateral orchidectomy (removal of testicles) in a vain attempt to assuage his sexual lust.
2. Karhausen, L. R., 'Mozart's 140 causes of death and 27 mental disorders', *British Medical Journal* 2010; 341: 1328–9.
3. Stuckenschmidt, H. H., *Arnold Schoenberg: His Life, World and Work*. Translated by Searle, H. John Calder, London, 1977, 491–6.
4. Kildea, P., *Benjamin Britten: A Life in the Twentieth Century*, Allen Lane, London, 2013, 532.
5. Petch, M. C., 'The Heart of Benjamin Britten', *Journal of the Royal Society of Medicine* 2014; 107: 339–41.

10

TUBERCULOSIS

Tuberculosis is caused by the bacterium *Mycobacterium tuberculosis*, identified and described by Robert Koch in 1882. Koch's findings showed that tuberculosis is an infectious disorder, although that it tended to afflict several members of the same family had long before strongly suggested that. Effective therapy came with the advent of antituberculous antibiotics in the second half of the twentieth century.

The soprano heroine in Verdi's *La Traviata* of 1853 is the courtesan Violetta Valéry, a character modelled on a celebrated real-life courtesan depicted in the play by Alexandre Dumas fils, *La Dame aux Camélias*. Verdi and his librettist Piave intended the action to be set contemporaneously and thus to evoke vivid realism. However, the authorities in Venice, where the première took place, would not permit the scandalous behaviour of the Parisian demi-monde to be seen as currently proceeding. Initially, therefore, the action was set much earlier: 'In and around Paris, about 1700'. Violetta is ill with tuberculosis of the lungs

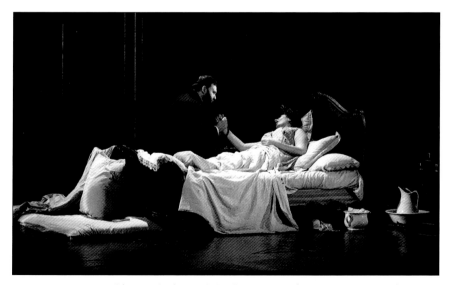

La Traviata: Dr Grenvil (James Platt) attends the dying Violetta (Anush Hovhannisyan). Scottish Opera 2017. Photo: Jane Hobson.

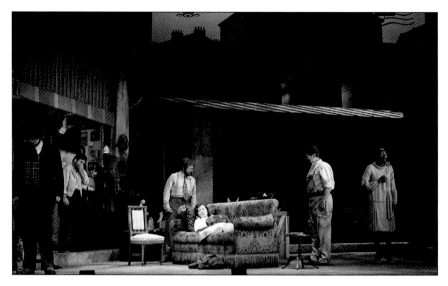

La Bohème (Puccini): The death of Mimì (Hye-Youn Lee). With her are Schaunard (Božidar Smiljanić), Rodolfo (Luis Gomes), Colline (Damien Pass), Marcello (David Stout), and Musetta (Jeanine De Bique). Note that the summoned doctor has failed to arrive. Scottish Opera 2017. Photo: Sally Jubb.

(pulmonary tuberculosis; phthisis; consumption). She is attended medically by the somewhat disreputable Doctor Grenvil, an habitué of the demi-monde sung by a bass. Doctor Grenvil can offer only comforting words and palliative medicines. Despite his care, Violetta dies.

The Parisian seamstress Mimì is a soprano character in two operas, each entitled *La Bohème* and composed respectively by Puccini (1896) and Leoncavallo (1897). Both were based on Henry Murger's novel *Scènes de la Vie de Bohème.* Like Violetta, Mimì is dying from pulmonary tuberculosis. By the date of these two operas the cause (but not the cure) of tuberculosis was known. Hence other characters might be expected to attempt the avoidance of infection and keep clear of Mimì's coughs. However, only an occasional director emphasizes this. In both operas a doctor is summoned, but in both Mimì dies before he arrives. Even so, as was seen in *La Traviata,* in the nineteenth century a doctor's efforts had at best a very marginal effect on survival.

UNSUCCESSFUL ANTI-TUBERCULOUS TREATMENT

As was noted above, drugs effective against tuberculosis became available only in the second half of the twentieth century. An interesting earlier attempt at treating tuberculosis was made in Giordano's opera *Mala Vita* of 1892 to a libretto by Nicola Daspuro. Amante (tenor) suffers from tuberculosis. In return for a cure he vows to Jesus to rescue a woman from a life of sin. This proposed course alarms and distresses his mistress Amalia (mezzo-soprano). Amante selects for his therapeutic purposes the aptly named local prostitute Cristina (soprano), to whom he proposes marriage. Amalia vainly attempts to bribe Cristina into giving up the marriage, then equally unsuccessfully threatens her with a knife. Amante, however, is more easily scared. Amalia readily intimidates him and he quickly gives way, declares once more his love for her and abandons Cristina. Cristina returns to her old dissolute life. The still ailing Amante goes back to carousing with his cronies. Perhaps surprisingly the opera was poorly received in Italy, where the subject matter was apparently perceived as shockingly sacrilegious.

WEBER'S AND CHEKHOV'S TUBERCULOSIS

A very distinguished composer succumbed to this disease. Carl Maria von Weber (1786–1826) was a major figure in the early development of German romantic opera. His influence on Wagner was clear and was acknowledged. Weber died in London in 1826 while supervising an acclaimed production of *Oberon*, his last opera. Post-mortem examination confirmed extensive tuberculous disease of the lungs. As was noted on page 8, the writer Anton Chekhov also died from pulmonary tuberculosis.

11

LEPROSY

Leprosy, also known as Hansen's disease, is a consequence of long-term infection with *Mycobacterium leprae*, a bacterium related to that causing tuberculosis. Infection can remain symptomless for as long as five to twenty years, before causing granulomatous lesions of nerves, respiratory tract, skin, and eyes. Pain sensation may disappear, leading to repeated initially unnoticed injury or infection, with the consequent loss of parts of extremities. Eyesight can be impaired. Skin lesions are disfiguring. Leprosy has since antiquity been known to be transmissible. Although not especially contagious, it is spread via long-term continual contact with infected persons living together, usually in poor conditions. The disease once carried social stigma, with lepers being often segregated in leper colonies. In public they might be required to advertise their presence by ringing a warning bell, and by crying out 'Unclean'. Leprosy is now responsive to antibiotic treatment.

The Moon and Sixpence of 1957 is an opera in three acts by John Gardner to a libretto by Patrick Terry after the novel of the same title by W. Somerset Maugham. Charles Strickland (bass-baritone) is a prosperous London stockbroker who suddenly decides to become an artistic painter. He abandons his fortune, sacrifices and exploits his family and friends, and neglects his own well-being. He travels to Tahiti where his creativity blossoms. He then unfortunately contracts leprosy. Despite the attentions of Dr Coutras (bass) and of his devoted native mistress Ata (soprano), he goes blind and dies.

Dalgerie, a tragic opera in one act, was composed in 1959 by James Penberthy to a libretto by Mary Durack after her novel *Keep Him My Country*. Dalgerie (soprano) is an Australian aboriginal woman with leprosy. She is forbidden by tribal law to marry her white lover Stan (baritone). Dalgerie performs magic love rituals to ensure that 'though they may be parted in life, their spirits can unite in death'. At their final meeting she reassures Stan that they will be reunited, then dies in his arms. Penberthy's score evokes mystical and melancholic aspects of the Australian outback via rhythms and melodies taken from aboriginal music.

Dalgerie has the distinction of being the very first opera to be performed at the newly built Sydney Opera House, on 23 July 1973.

Olivier Messiaen composed the opera *Saint François d'Assise* (St Francis of Assisi) of 1983 to his own libretto. In Act I St Francis (baritone) meets a Leper (tenor) who is in great physical and spiritual distress. St Francis tries to teach the Leper acceptance, but is rejected. Then an Angel (soprano) appears and sings that God is love. St Francis realizes that he has been insufficiently charitable. He embraces the Leper and so effects a miraculous cure. The tattered delirious patient is transformed back to elegant normality.

12

CHOLERA

Cholera results from infection of the bowel by the bacterium *Vibrio cholerae*. The most frequent cause is the drinking of polluted water. There follows usually severe diarrhoea and vomiting, symptoms not readily suitable for portrayal on stage. Hardly surprisingly, operatic depiction of cholera has been muted.

In Alban Berg's opera *Lulu* of 1935, the soprano Lulu of the title role is imprisoned for the murder of her third husband, Dr Schön (baritone). Lulu's lesbian admirer Countess Geschwitz (mezzo-soprano) deliberately infects Lulu with cholera and then self-sacrificingly changes places with her secretly when Lulu is admitted to hospital. The escaped Lulu is noticeably thin and weak, the only features of the disease to be shown on stage.

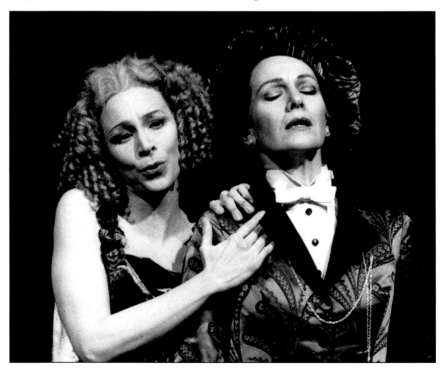

Lulu: The lesbian Countess Geschwitz (Delia Wallis, right) infects Lulu (Beverly Morgan) with cholera. Scottish Opera 1987. Photo: Eric Thorburn.

The opera *Lanzelot* by Paul Dessau was composed to a libretto by Heiner Müller and Ginka Cholakowa after the fairy-tale *Der Drache* (*The Dragon*) by Hans Christian Andersen and Yevgeni Schwartz. It was first performed in 1969. This work is of especial interest in that it depicts a public health approach by purifying the polluted source of the disease. A dragon (bass) has helped to eliminate an epidemic of cholera in a town by breathing fire to boil the infected water. In return, however, the dragon demands the annual payment of a young maiden. Lanzelot (baritone) proposes to fight the dragon and so save Elsa (soprano), the latest intended victim. Lanzelot slays the dragon. But then the Bürgermeister (tenor) proclaims himself president and demands Elsa's hand in marriage. Happily the people rise up, depose the president, and celebrate their new-found freedom from both cholera and dragon. Lanzelot gets his girl.

Benjamin Britten's last opera, *Death in Venice* of 1973, is to a libretto by Myfanwy Piper after the novella by the German writer Thomas Mann, *Der Tod in Venedig* of 1912. Gustav von Aschenbach (tenor) is a distinguished writer in his late fifties. A widower, he is a man dedicated to his art, disciplined and ascetic to the point of severity. Aschenbach takes a holiday in Venice. There he sees, and from a distance falls in love with, a beautiful Polish youth, Tadzio (silent).

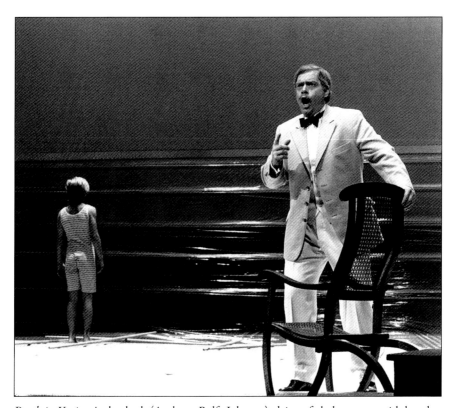

Death in Venice: Aschenbach (Anthony Rolfe Johnson), dying of cholera, gazes with hopeless yearning on the beautiful youth Tadzio (Craig Fraser). Scottish Opera 1983. Photo: Lewis Segal.

Albeit Aschenbach makes several attempts, at no stage can he bring himself to speak to the boy. An epidemic of cholera breaks out in Venice. For a time the authorities manage to keep this secret, but the information leaks out, and holidaymakers begin to leave. On the day that Tadzio is due to depart with his family Aschenbach, sitting in a deck chair on the beach, is admiring him longingly. Aschenbach dies. The cause of Aschenbach's death is usually taken to be cholera. If so, the symptoms he displays in the opera are remarkably subdued. As noted on page 114, Ober (among others) has speculated on the alternative possibility of a fatal cardiac arrhythmia.

13

PLAGUE

In strict medical terminology, plague is a disease caused by infection with the bacillus *Yersinia pestis*, an organism nowadays readily eliminated by antibiotics. *Yersinia pestis* was almost certainly responsible for the Black Death, which swept across Europe in the fourteenth century. However, in opera as elsewhere, the term 'plague' is often employed less exactly to denote any severe affliction of whole populations. Of the biblical ten plagues of ancient Egypt, only the sixth (boils) and the tenth (death of the firstborn) involved human disease; neither suggests *Yersinia* infection.

The ancient Greek dramatist Sophocles wrote a trilogy of plays based on the Oedipus legend, which is summarised in Chapter 25. Numerous operas have been derived from that trilogy. These include *Oedipus at Colonus* (1786) by Sacchini to a libretto by Guillard; Rossini's unpublished *Oedipus at Colonus* (1816); Stravinsky's *Oedipus Rex* (1927) to a libretto by Cocteau; Enescu's *Oedipe* (1936) to a libretto by Fleg; Partch's *Oedipus* (1952) to his own libretto; Orff's *Oedipus der Tyrann* (1959) to a German translation by Hölderlin; Rihm's *Oedipus* (1987) to his own text after Hölderlin; and Julian Anderson's *Thebans* (2014) to a libretto by Frank McGuinness. Additionally, Purcell in 1692 composed music for a play, *Oedipus*, by Dryden and Lees. All involve a plague imposed by the gods on Thebes because of the sins of patricide and incest committed by King Oedipus. The identity of the plague is not specified in the drama. However, Kousoulis *et al.*,[1] from a detailed analysis of the plays by Sophocles, and a systematic review of historical data, suggest that this could have been an epidemic of brucellosis, caused by the bacillus *Brucella abortus,* spread to the population from infected cattle. In Mark-Anthony Turnage's opera *Greek* of 1988 the legend was updated to London's East End in the late twentieth century; the 'plague' there was greed and avarice under Margaret Thatcher's government.

There are nevertheless several operas which involve genuine plague. *Guido et Ginevra* or *The Plague of Florence* (1838) was composed by Fromental Halévy to a libretto by Scribe. Ginevra (soprano), daughter of Cosimo dei Medici (bass), collapses during her marriage ceremony to the Duke of Ferrara (bass). It is assumed that she is a victim of the plague currently ravaging Florence and she is interred in the Medici vault. She then recovers consciousness, but everywhere she goes in the plague-ridden city she is shunned, until a young sculptor, Guido (tenor), gives her shelter. The two fall in love. Cosimo is eventually persuaded to approve his daughter's marriage to Guido.

Two operas were composed to Alessandro Manzoni's novel *I Promessi Sposi* (*The Betrothed*): Ponchielli's to an anonymous libretto (1856) and Petrella's to a libretto by Ghislanzoni (1869). Both tell the same tale. Don Rodrigo (baritone) is stricken with the plague which is raging in Florence. He sends for his personal physician. Then seeing the *monatti*, stretcher-bearers appointed for the dying, arriving instead, he shoots himself.

Richard Rodney Bennett's opera *The Mines of Sulphur* to a libretto by Beverley Cross, dates from 1965. The action takes place in a lonely manor house in the West of England in the eighteenth century. A trio of ruffians (tenor, baritone and mezzo-soprano) break in, murder the owner (bass-baritone) and proceed to plunder the household. They are then surprised by a troupe of touring actors seeking shelter for the night. The players give an impromptu performance of their latest drama, *The Mines of Sulphur*, in the course of which the actress Jenny (soprano) faints. Jenny is carried upstairs, where the body of the murdered landlord is discovered. The evil trio prepare to imprison the actors in the cellar then make their escape. But the ailing Jenny reveals the dreadful truth that there can be no escape; she is infected with the plague. Although the libretto is not explicit, the dramatic context makes clear that the infecting organism here is highly virulent. This can be taken to be an instance of genuine plague.

---

1. Kousoulis A. A., Economopoulos K. P., Poulakou-Rebelaku E., Androutsos G., Tsiodras S. 'The Plague of Thebes, a Historical Epidemic in Sophocles' *Oedipus Rex*, *Emerging Infectious Diseases* 2012; 18: 153–7.

RABIES

Rabies is a disease of severe inflammation of the brain consequent upon infection with one of the group of lyssaviruses. Almost always it results from a bite or scratch by an infected animal, most often a dog. The incubation time from infection to symptoms can vary from one week to three months, depending on the site of the initial lesion. This is because the virus must travel up the peripheral nerves to reach the brain. The features of rabies are extremely distressing, including excitement, confusion, fear or hatred of water, loss of consciousness, uncontrolled and often violent movements, and paralysis. The disease can be diagnosed only when symptoms appear. Death almost always ensues.

El Rey Que Rabió (*The King Who Was Rabid*) of 1891 is a zarzuela by Ruperto Chapi to a libretto by Miguel Ramos Carrion and Vital Aza. A zarzuela is a particularly Spanish operatic genre in which singing is interspersed with passages of spoken dialogue and dancing. The young King (soprano) is, in disguise, touring to inspect his realm. Jeremías (tenor) is bitten by a dog and then mistaken for the King. There is uncertainty whether or not the dog is rabid. A huddle of doctors is swiftly convened but despite protracted argument reaches no decision. Fortunately the dog turns out not be infected. No one develops rabies and all ends happily.

The opera *Love and Other Demons* of 2008 was by the Hungarian composer Péter Eötvös to a libretto by Kornél Hamvai after the 1994 novel *Of Love and Other Demons* by Gabriel Garcia Márquez. The twelve-year-old Sierva Maria (soprano) is bitten by a dog subsequently found to be infected with rabies. There ensues an anxious period of uncertainty concerning the outcome. This is suddenly interrupted by the Bishop (bass), who decides that exorcism of possible demons may help. Catastrophically, as the Bishop determinedly pursues exorcism, Sierva Maria suffers a convulsion and dies. Whether or not this is a consequence of rabies is left unclear.

15

HUMAN IMMUNODEFICIENCY VIRUS (HIV) INFECTION AND ACQUIRED IMMUNODEFICIENCY SYNDROME (AIDS)

Acquired immunodeficiency syndrome (AIDS) was first recognised in the 1980s. An initial infection with the human immunodeficiency virus (HIV) may pass unnoticed or cause a brief influenza-like illness. There follows a symptomless period of months or years before progressive interference with the immune system results in a predisposition to common infections such as tuberculosis and to develop tumours that would be suppressed in a person with normal immune processes. These late features are referred to as acquired immunodeficiency syndrome (AIDS). AIDS affects mainly young adults. A major means of HIV transmission is unprotected sex, including anal or oral sex. There is a strongly perceived association between AIDS and male homosexual behaviour with consequent social stigma. Another major hazard is the use of contaminated syringes by drug addicts. There is at present no cure, although antiretroviral treatment can slow the course of the disease, and may provide a near-normal life expectancy. Pre-exposure prophylaxis (PrEP) is the use of antiviral drugs as a preventive measure. The drug combination emtricitabine tenofovir disopraxil fumarate has been employed with some success with this approach in persons at high risk.

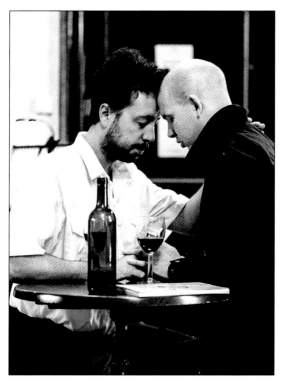

Love Speaks: The male homosexual pair (Douglas Nairne and Kenny Reid). NOISE 2018. Photo: Kris Kesiak.

AIDS first appeared operatically in a composition based on Tony Kushner's 1991 play *Angels in America: A Gay Fantasia on National Themes*. This play is a complex, often metaphorical and symbolic study of AIDS and homosexuality in the USA in the 1980s. The two parts of the play, which are presentable separately, are subtitled *Millennium Approaches* and *Perestroika*. The convolutions of the plot of *Angels in America* defy ready précis and are not easily comprehended even at performance. Five male homosexuals, Prior, Louis, Joe, Roy, and Belize, are variously suffering from HIV infection and AIDS. Prior additionally is seeing angels and receiving advice from heavenly voices. Joe's wife Harper is agoraphobic and experiencing drug-induced hallucinations. Roy is stealing antiviral medicines intended for a trial of AIDS therapy. The action becomes progressively more labyrinthine, with Prior getting increasingly clamant instructions from divine prompters. Part II and thus the overall play concludes with Prior addressing the audience directly, and assuring them that God's 'Great Work' will continue.

In 2004 the play was adapted by the Hungarian composer Péter Eötvös as the opera *Angels in America*. The opera is based on both parts of the original play, reworked and condensed so as to run for just two and a half hours. Eötvös has said, 'I put less emphasis on the political line than Kushner ... I rather focus on the passionate relationships, on the highly dramatic suspense of the wonderful text, on the permanently uncertain state of the visions.'

The composer Kevin O'Reilly's opera *Love Speaks*, to a libretto by Jenny Knotts, is a 15-minute work given by NOISE (New Opera In Scotland Events). It had its first performance in August 2018 in one of the Victorian rooms at Sloans, Glasgow's oldest bar and restaurant. The cast of two sopranos, tenor and baritone plus a speaking actress is accompanied by a chamber orchestra comprising piano, violin, cello, accordion and percussion. The setting, appropriately for the première, is a bar. The work opens with the actress, as barmaid, addressing the audience directly, and informing them that the opera was commissioned to celebrate the Scottish Government's decision to have PrEP available on prescription to persons at risk of HIV infection. Her enunciation of 'emtricitabine tenofovir disopraxil fumarate' in a broad Glasgow accent is unfailingly uproarious. The simple plot is of two homosexual pairs becoming acquainted, then falling in love. The opening section, in which the characters tentatively reach out to each other, is to rhythmically jagged music, with stressed vocal syllables making up the complex full chemical wording of the PrEP. Then, as the couples fall in love, both music and text become smoothly lyrical.

Although in outline the libretto appeared unpromisingly banal, this very short opera came across as both musically and dramatically convincing, and was well received.

16

DISEASES OF THE EYE

Real-life ophthalmologists, specialists in diseases of the eye, suffer a rather poor reputation in musical circles. Johann Sebastian Bach died in 1750 apparently from the consequences of a botched operation for cataract. The same quack ophthalmologist as dealt with Bach, John 'Chevalier' Taylor, failed also in 1758 to deal properly with Handel's cataracts. Neither setback seems to have inhibited Taylor from boasting of his famous patients. Liszt was another composer who suffered from cataracts. He was advised by his ophthalmologist, Dr Gräfe, to undergo operation, but Liszt was apparently so fearful that he repeatedly deferred the surgery and died still with his cataracts. An unsuccessful cataract operation is believed to have hastened Glyndebourne founder John Christie's death in 1962.[1] Operatic ophthalmologists by contrast have often, but not always, performed much better.

In Gyrowetz's *Der Augenarzt* of 1811 to a libretto by Johann Emanuel Veith, the ophthalmologist Berg (tenor) operates successfully. He restores the sight of Philipp and Wilhelmine (both soprano) who have been blind from birth.

In Tchaikovsky's *Iolanta* of 1892 to a libretto by his brother Modest, the Princess Iolanta (soprano) has likewise been blind from birth. She is cured after an operation by Ibn-Hakia (baritone).

Less successful is the Egyptian ophthalmologist Ktesiphar in d'Albert's *Die Toten Augen* of 1916 to a text by Hans Heinz Ewers and Marc Henry. Myrtocle (soprano) is yet another who has been blind from birth. She longs to see her husband Arcesius (baritone), who she believes to be as handsome as Apollo. As she has been blind from birth it is difficult to understand what concept she has of this. Arcesius is in fact ugly and mis-shapen. Nevertheless this is opera and hence for dramatic reasons her belief and hopes must be accommodated. Unlike Berg and Ibn-Hakia, the therapeutic efforts of Ktesiphar unfortunately fail, but he is rescued by Jesus (sung by an off-stage tenor) and Myrtocle is granted sight. A man as handsome as Apollo does indeed appear, but it is Galba (tenor), her husband's friend, who has loved her for years. Arcesius kills Galba and Myrtocle blinds herself again by staring at the sun.

Medically it is disappointing that in none of these operas are details provided of the optic pathology.

---

1.   Norwich, J. J., *Fifty Years of Glyndebourne*, Jonathan Cape, London, 1985, p. 86.

17

LOSS OF VOICE

In opera, vocal impairment or loss is nearly always inadvertent, the consequence of a severe cold. This is the dread of singers and the joy of their covers or understudies. Occasionally, however, loss of voice is purposely written into a libretto.

In Donizetti's *Il Campanello di Notte* of 1836 (see also page 58 and Chapter 28) one of the subterfuges adopted by Enrico (baritone) is to pose as a singer who has lost his voice. Demanding a therapeutic prescription, he rings the night bell of the pharmacy, requiring his formal rival in love, the pharmacist Don Annibale Pistacchio (bass), to leave his bed and his bride.

Dvořák's *Rusalka* of 1901 was composed to a libretto by Jaroslav Kapil. The water nymph Rusalka is sung by the *prima donna* soprano who must therefore be taken to be the pre-eminent singer. Rusalka falls in love with the Prince (tenor)

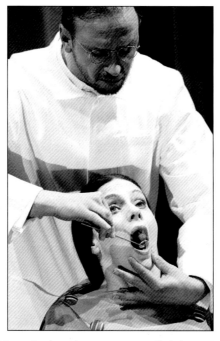

Rusalka: A doctor (Martin Lindinger) investigates Rusalka's (Anne Sophie Duprels) Act II muteness. Scottish Opera 2016. Photo: James Glossop.

but in order to join him she must assume human form. This she does, under the condition that she remains mute; hence Rusalka, despite being played by the leading soprano, does not sing for most of Act II. The Prince, however, rejects her and sadly she returns to her aquatic habitat, where because of her mortal ambitions she is then spurned by her sister nymphs. In Act III the Prince has a change of heart and pursues her. Rusalka is no longer silent, and there is glorious singing. Finally the pair embrace, kiss, and sink together into a watery grave.

A prominent non-medical instance of operatic voice loss is that of the baritone Papageno in Mozart's *The Magic Flute*. His lips are padlocked by the Three Ladies (two sopranos, one mezzo-soprano) as a punishment for boastful mendacity.

Aside from *The Magic Flute* and Papageno, probably the most famous of all operas with an important silent role is Auber's *La Muette de Portici* of 1828 to a libretto by Scribe and Delavigne. This deals with the unsuccessful 1647 Neapolitan rebellion against Spanish rule. The Muette (mute) of the title is Fenella, played by a dancer. Her brother Masaniello (tenor) is leader of the revolt. Fenella is seduced and then abandoned by Alphonse (tenor), son of the Spanish Viceroy of Naples. She is briefly imprisoned by the Viceroy. Masaniello incites rebellion but then loses control of events and is horrified at the slaughter and destruction. He loses his reason and has a notable mad scene. He is then murdered by his own people. The rebellion is brutally put down, Alphonse, the Viceroy's son, is hailed as victor, and Fenella, overcome with grief, kills herself by jumping into a flow of lava from the eruption of Vesuvius.

This opera is especially notable as being the very first of the Parisian *grand opéra* genre. All the ingredients are there: a historical subject; five acts; extensive ballet; a mad scene; and the concluding spectacle of a volcanic eruption.

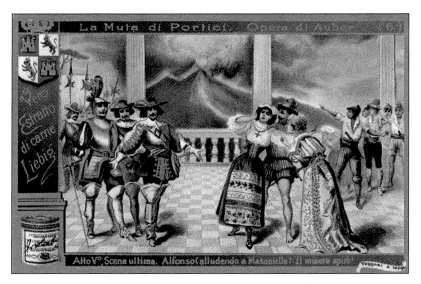

La Muette de Portici: Illustration of an Italian production showing the final scene with the eruption of Vesuvius. Private Collection/Look and Learn/Rosenberg Collection/Bridgeman Images.

HEART DISEASE

A PROLAPSED MITRAL VALVE

Offenbach's opera *The Tales of Hoffmann* was composed to a libretto by Barbier based on an 1851 play by Barbier and Carré. This was Offenbach's last opera; he died while it was in rehearsal for its first performance, which took place in Paris in 1881. The opera depicts a series of episodes in the life of the real-life writer and composer E. T. A. Hoffmann, who lived from 1776 to 1822. In the opera the role of Hoffmann is sung by a tenor.

A cardiac problem is encountered in one episode. Hoffmann is in love with the nineteen-year-old Antonia (soprano), the daughter of Crespel (bass). Antonia has inherited a heart complaint from her mother, a singer who died young from that disorder and whose portrait hangs on the wall. Although Antonia has a beautiful voice, there are fears that singing may endanger her life, and her father forbids it. Crespel blames inappropriate treatment advised by her physician Dr Miracle (baritone) to have been responsible for his wife's death, and he wishes Dr Miracle to have no involvement in the treatment of the daughter. Dr Miracle is unquestionably thoroughly evil. He comments on the sinister red patches that appear on Antonia's cheeks when she sings. He takes her pulse and describes fast irregular beating. Dr Miracle surprises Antonia when she is alone and urges her to sing, using witchcraft to conjure up the ghost of her dead mother, a mezzo-soprano. Dr Miracle seizes a violin and leads them in a frantic trio. Antonia collapses to the floor. Crespel and Hoffmann rush desperately in, but the Doctor pronounces Antonia to be dead.

The nature of the heart complaint suffered by mother and daughter has attracted a good deal of medical interest and speculation over the years. Dr Leonard Dauber,[1] considering several possibilities, concluded that probably both Antonia and her mother suffered from prolapse of the mitral valve of the heart, one of several varieties of that disease, this particular form inherited as an autosomal dominant condition, and frequently associated with a frail physique. Patients may complain of shortness of breath or exertion and they are readily fatigued. They can have rapid and often irregular beating of the heart, such disturbance of the heart rhythm being provoked by increases in circulating adrenaline as can be caused by excitement of any kind. Sudden death can readily occur. According to Dr Dauber, Antonia should have been treated with a beta-adrenergic blocking drug (a beta-blocker) such as propranolol, which would have prevented the harmful effects of raised blood levels of adrenaline on the heart rhythm, the excess adrenaline evoked in this instance by the excitement of singing. However, beta-blocking drugs were not available in Hoffmann's time, being developed by Sir James Black only in the 1960s. If Antonia had taken a beta-blocker she could probably have sung without restriction, although perhaps rather placidly. Against that, of course, we should have been deprived of a good story and a dramatic operatic portrayal.

Interestingly, and surprisingly, both Ober[2] and the Hutcheons[3] take Antonia's disease not to be cardiac, but pulmonary tuberculosis. Goldovsky more vaguely suggests an inherited 'weakness of the lungs'.[4] In this all of them are, I consider, mistaken.

HEART TRANSPLANTATION

Hans Pfitzner's opera *Das Herz* (*The Heart*) to a libretto by Hans Mahner-Mons was first staged in 1931. Dr Daniel Athanasius (baritone) is called upon to treat the dying Prince Tancred (spoken). Athanasius makes a sacrilegious pact with the demon Asmodi (tenor). Athanasius is granted possession for one year of a heart taken from a living person. The heart must then after a year pass to Asmodi. Athanasius thus acquires a heart, implants the heart into Prince Tancred and restores him to health. But then, at the first anniversary celebrations of the Prince's recovery, Asmodi reappears and demands to be given the heart. If the Prince is to be saved, Athanasius must enter into a second profane contract, and a second heart will be taken from a healthy victim. The donor demanded by Asmodi is Helge (soprano), the wife of Athanasius. The doctor refuses this dreadful behest. Prince Tancred dies. The life of Dr Athanasius is also forfeited, but his soul is saved.

With the advent of *Regietheater*, directors began to mount operatic productions that deviated, often markedly, from the original stage directions. Thus, when heart transplant surgery became possible in the 1960s it was soon apparent that *Das Herz* could convincingly be updated to a contemporary clinical setting. Particularly relevant was the often transient survival of early heart transplants. In 1993 Peter P. Pachl directed a production of *Das Herz* at Rudolstadt, Germany in which the action was set in a modern hospital. Two characters, in the original called First and Second Executioner, became First and Second Assistant Physician.

A futile attempt at cardiac transplantation is made in the opera *Artémis*, composed in 1898 by Alberto Nepomuceno to a libretto by Coelo Neto. Helio (tenor), a sculptor, falls in love with a statue of the goddess Artemis of his own creation. He tears out the heart of his daughter Delia with the intention of imparting life to the statue. He fails. Delia dies and the statue remains inert.

ANGINA PECTORIS

Cardiac angina (angina pectoris) results from pathological narrowing of the coronary arteries, the arteries supplying the heart muscle. On exercise, or with excitement, when cardiac output is increased, insufficient blood reaches the heart muscle, leading to pain (angina), usually in the central chest or throat.

Angina appears surprisingly rarely in opera. It does occur in *Mourning Becomes Electra* of 1967, composed by Marvin David Levy to a libretto by Henry Butler after Eugene O'Neill's trilogy of plays. Christine (soprano) deliberately confesses to her husband Ezra (bass) that she is having an illicit affair with the sea-captain Adam (baritone) so as to provoke an attack of angina, which it does. Then, instead of his medicine, she gives Ezra poison, and kills him.

The death of the Tsar Boris (bass or baritone) at the end of Mussorgsky's *Boris Godunov* is usually taken to result from a heart attack caused by coronary artery disease. As is noted on page 116, the orchestral accompaniment vividly suggests this.

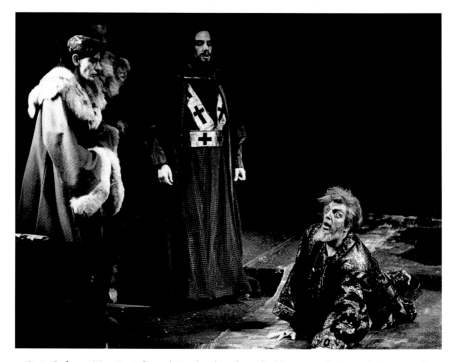

Boris Godunov: Tsar Boris (Joseph Rouleau) suffers a fatal heart attack. Scottish Opera 1968.

WAGNER'S ANGINA

The composer Richard Wagner suffered from angina pectoris over the last months of his life. He died probably from coronary thrombosis following a severe attack on 13 February 1883.

1. Dauber, L. G., 'Death in Opera: A Case Study', *American Journal of Cardiology* 1992; 70: 838–40.
2. Ober, W. B., 'Operatic "Doctors"', *The Practitioner* 1976; 216: 110–16.
3. Hutcheon, L., and Hutcheon, M., *Opera: Desire, Disease, Death*, University of Nebraska Press, Lincoln, USA, 1996, 30–7.
4. Goldovsky, B., 'Some Medical Matters in Operatic Literature', *Cleveland Clinic Quarterly* 1986; 53: 39–43.

19

GASTROINTESTINAL ABNORMALITIES AND OTHER PHENOMENA

Diseases of the digestive system and bowels are largely unsuitable for operatic depiction. As noted in Chapter 12, presentation of the features of cholera are for that reason in opera usually suppressed into virtual absence. There are, however, some rare but interesting exceptions. In Haydn's *The Apothecary* of 1768 to a libretto by Goldoni, the apprentice Mengoni (tenor) sings the praises of a good purgative: 'Per quel che la mal stomacho'. In Donizetti's *Il Campanello di Notte* (see also page 52 and Chapter 28) a (fictional) patient has seven intestinal fistulae plus flatulence.

Richard Strauss's *Feuersnot (Fire-Famine)* started out well but then suffered bowdlerization. This opera, dating from 1901, was to a libretto by Ernst von Wolzogen, he of the Berlin Überbrettl cabaret (see page 16). The topic selected by Strauss was an episode from an ancient Dutch tale. A young man, spurned in love by a haughty maiden, calls a malediction on the town. Every fire, lamp, hearth, and all is extinguished. This curse can be exorcized in only one way, and that a demanding one. The distraught citizens nevertheless agree. The proud and cruel girl is then made to undress completely and to kneel on a table. Suddenly a flame magically erupts from her anus and the townsfolk line up with their candles and light them from this unusual source. It takes many hours before all have fire.

Sadly, this potential *coup de théâtre* had to be excised from the opera and the plot modified. The beautiful maiden Diemut (soprano) entices Kunad (baritone) and pretends to welcome him to her upstairs room. The eager Kunad is hoisted upwards in a basket. But Diemut, fickle and devious, leaves him dangling mid-air out of reach of her balcony and then proceeds to mock and taunt him, to the delight and raucous jeering of the watching populace. Kunad, enraged, casts a spell on the town, and all its fires are extinguished. At this the distressed townsfolk call upon Diemut to surrender to this excellent young man and so lift the curse. Diemut relents, and takes Kunad up into her room. In darkness a beautiful orchestral passage signifies consummation of their union. There follows a moment of silence before every fire blazes once more.

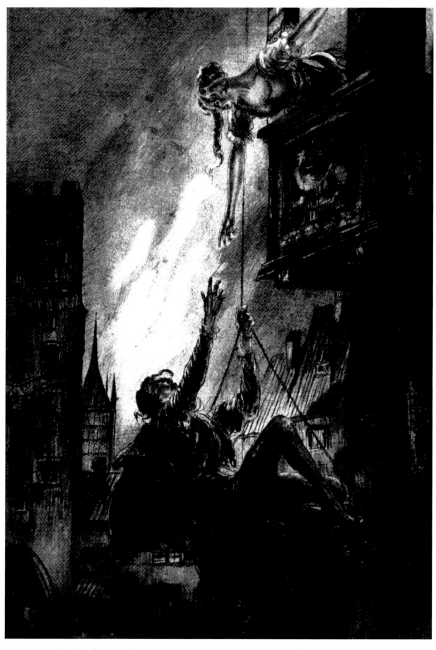

Feuersnot: The haughty maiden Diemut taunts and teases Kunrad, hanging mid-air in a basket. Etching by the Austrian artist Alois Kolb (1875–1942). Lebrecht Music Arts/Bridgeman Images.

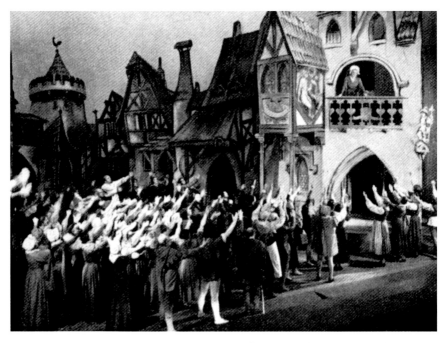

Feuersnot: The desperate townsfolk implore Diemut (Annie Krull) to help them lift the curse. Scene from the Dresden première, 1901. Lebrecht Music Arts/Bridgeman Images.

Various rumours, mostly of very dubious provenance, concern the genesis of *Feuersnot*. It has been put about that Richard Strauss, resentful at the failure of his first opera *Guntram*, took up the story as being so outrageous as to be a sure sensation. Yet Strauss could never have been so wildly optimistic as to suppose the text to be acceptable or that, even if it were, any soprano would consent to take on the role of Diemut, despite that being an unquestionable guarantor of fame. Even the final bowdlerized version was banned in Berlin on the Kaiser's orders as being too bawdy. But we can regret that the full original ancient yarn never took operatic shape.

20

STROKE

Stroke, sometimes also termed apoplexy, results from rupture or occlusion (usually by blood clotting) of an artery supplying part of the brain. Very common in real life, it is an affliction seen only rarely on the operatic stage.

In Rachmaninov's *The Miserly Knight* of 1906 to a text by Pushkin, the baritone of the title role is summoned to answer charges of non-support of his son, but then dies suddenly. The cause, we are informed, is apoplexy.

A much more interesting attack occurs in Verdi's *Nabucco* of 1842 to a libretto by Solera. In the second scene of Part II, the baritone Nabucco declares himself not only King but God. For this blasphemy a thunderbolt immediately strikes him down. Nabucco, however, does not die. After prolonged distracted disability, by the end of the opera, in the second scene of Part IV, he has made a full recovery. In the libretto this is attributed to his conversion to Judaism. In strictly medical terms, successful post-stroke rehabilitation seems more likely.

PIAVE'S STROKE

A particularly distressing real-life instance of stroke was that suffered by the librettist Francesco Piave (1810–76). Piave wrote over sixty opera libretti, including ten for Verdi (*Ernani*, *I Due Foscari*, *Attila*, *Macbeth*, *Il Corsaro*, *Stiffelio*, *Rigoletto*, *La Traviata*, *Simon Boccanegra*, and *La Forza del Destino*). Piave was also a tactfully skilled negotiator and accomplished stage manager. Verdi undoubtedly bullied Piave mercilessly but seemed always to retain his loyalty. In 1867 Piave had a severe stroke which left him paralysed and speechless. He survived in this pitiful state for another eight years, over which time Verdi nobly repaid his debt by financially supporting him, together with his wife and daughter. The composer later also paid Piave's funeral expenses.

21

VISUAL AGNOSIA

Visual agnosia is a rare disorder resulting from damage to the parts of the brain responsible for the interpretation of visual stimuli. The patient can see, but is unable to recognise, or to find sense in, what is seen. Michael Nyman's opera of 1986, *The Man Who Mistook His Wife for a Hat*, to a libretto by Christopher Rawlence, is based on a true account of a case under the care of the neurological physician Dr Oliver Sacks.[1]

The patient, Mr P, a baritone, is a professional singer of classical music. The opinion of Dr S (tenor) is sought because of behavioural peculiarities displayed by Mr P. While clearly not demented, he often fails to recognise his singing students, although he does identify them when he hears them speak. On his way to a recent concert he found himself unable to interpret a street map. He then asked a parking meter to direct him. When the parking meter remained silent he addressed his enquiries to a pillar box.

At the consultation with Dr S, as the patient and his wife are leaving, she guides him towards the hat rack. Mr P then reaches out for her head, mistaking it for his hat. Dr S realises that the problem is visual agnosia. The patient is shown a rose. He describes what he sees in these terms:

> Six inches in length,
> Convoluted red form,
> With a linear green attachment.

Yet these observations, factually correct, convey nothing coherent to him. Only when he is asked to smell it does he identify the object as a rose.

It transpires that Mr P has found that hummed tunes, especially by one of his favourite composers, Schumann, can help him coordinate simple everyday tasks, such as eating a meal, which would otherwise, because of his inability to make cognitive visual judgement, be almost impossible. Dr S encourages Mr P to cultivate even more the coherence that, as he already discovered for himself, music can provide, and to utilize those talents to the utmost.

This is a true story. It is notable that, as is discussed in Chapter 33, St Louis found the relationship established here between doctor and patient to be one of the most commendable in opera.

1.   Sacks, O., *The Man Who Mistook His Wife for a Hat*, Picador, London, 1986.

EPILEPSY

Epilepsy is a disorder of brain function which occurs in two principal varieties. Minor (petit mal) epilepsy is characterised by transient losses of concentration or consciousness lasting usually for a few moments only and often passing unnoticed by both the patient and companions. It is not a condition which is suitable for operatic portrayal. Major (grand mal) epilepsy is more spectacular. The patient suffers a convulsive fit, losing consciousness and collapsing to the ground. Incontinence of urine or faeces is not unusual. Several minutes may elapse before consciousness is regained. A much rarer variety, temporal lobe epilepsy, makes at least one striking appearance in opera.

MAJOR EPILEPSY

Verdi's *Otello* of 1887 was composed to a libretto by Arrigo Boito after Shakespeare's play. At the end of Act III, Otello (tenor) suffers a major (grand mal) epileptic fit. As the offstage chorus acclaims Otello as the 'Lion of Venice', Iago (baritone) places one foot on Otello's unconscious prostrate form and contemptuously shouts 'Ecco il Leone!' ('Behold the Lion!'). This is a *coup de théâtre* giving a vivid conclusion to the act. Interestingly, Francesco Berio di Salsa, the librettist of Rossini's 1816 *Otello*, provided several variant texts, none of which however features Otello's epileptic fit.

The opera *The Idiot* of 1970 by Luciano Chailly was composed to a libretto by Gilberto Loverso after the novel by Dostoyevsky. Prince Myskin (tenor), naive, temperamentally fragile, and epileptic, is nicknamed 'The Idiot'. Myskin's pervasive epilepsy emphasizes his inability to adjust to the harrowing events he must endure. Myskin is a suitor for the hand of Nastasia (mezzo-soprano). His rival is Prince Rogozin (baritone). Nastasia initially elopes with Rogozin but then leaves him, later becoming engaged to Myskin. Then on the wedding day Nastasia is once more carried off by Rogozin, at whose hand she meets her death. The mentally unstable epileptic Myskin cannot cope with all this, and the opera ends with his wild ravings.

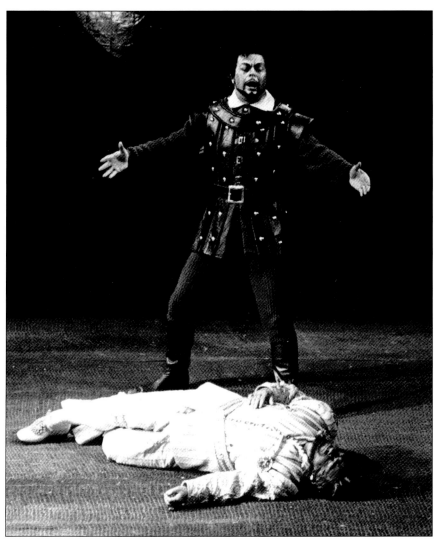

Otello (Verdi): Iago (Peter Glossop) stands over the stricken epileptic Otello (Charles Craig).
Scottish Opera 1972. Photo: Bob Anderson.

TEMPORAL LOBE EPILEPSY

Benjamin Britten composed his opera *The Turn of the Screw* in 1954 to a libretto by
Myfanwy Piper after the story of 1898 by Henry James. The Governess (soprano)
has been placed in sole charge of two orphan children, Miles (treble) and Flora
(soprano), at a remote country house. She begins to experience visions of a former
governess, Miss Jessel (soprano), and a former manservant, Peter Quint (tenor).
These two had previously exerted an evil influence on the children; both are now
dead.

The neurological physician Purdon Martin pointed out[1] that although Henry James did not state this in his story, he was describing in the Governess attacks of temporal lobe epilepsy. This condition results from an abnormality of the temporal lobe of the brain and is characterised by often vivid hallucinations or dreams. Temporal lobe epilepsy was first described by the neurologist Hughlings Jackson and reported in the journal *Brain*. In his article, Martin speculates on how Henry James could have learned of this unusual, but very dramatic, illness. The publisher of *Brain* was Frederick Macmillan, who was also Henry James's publisher. Martin wonders if Macmillan, knowing of James's great interest in matters eerie, could have told him about temporal lobe epilepsy.

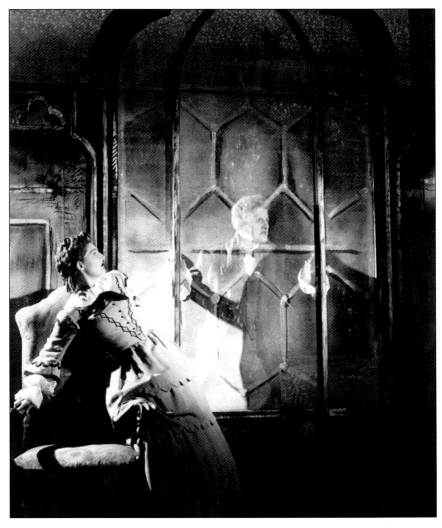

The Turn of the Screw: The epileptic Governess (Jennifer Vyvyan) sees an apparition of the dead Peter Quint (Peter Pears). English Opera Group 1954. Denis de Marney/Boosey and Hawkes Collection/ArenaPAL.

One might reflect on whether the manifestations seen by Joan of Arc in Verdi's *Giovanna d'Arco* and Tchaikovsky's *The Maid of Orléans* are a consequence of temporal lobe epilepsy. Of course, both operas are derived from Schiller's play, which antedated the work of Hughlings Jackson.

1. Martin, J. P., 'Neurology in Fiction: *The Turn of the Screw*', *British Medical Journal* 1973; 4: 717–21.

23

SOMNAMBULISM

Somnambulism is a sleep disorder characterised by combined sleeping and wakefulness. Typically it occurs in the first third of the night. In an attack the patient performs apparently unconscious activities that are more usually undertaken in full consciousness. These may comprise simply sitting up in bed, or walking around the room, although more complex, potentially hazardous, behaviour such as cooking, driving, or even attempted homicide can occur. The eyes are usually open but expressionless. An episode can last for 30 minutes or even longer. Typically, but not invariably, the patient has no subsequent memory of the sleepwalking events.

Sleepwalking has obvious appeal as a dramatic device in opera. Michele Carafa's *Il Sonnambulo* of 1824 was to a libretto by Romani. Ernesto (bass) has become Duke of Scilla by murdering his elder brother Ansaldo and has cast guilt for the crime onto the innocent courtier Adolfo. But Ernesto is oppressed by remorse. Every night at 3am, the hour he killed his brother, he sleepwalks around the castle 'with motionless eyes'. Then, one night, before horrified onlookers, he inadvertently confesses his crime: 'As long as I live, every time I hear the castle's bell ring at this terrible hour, I will hear Ansaldo's last cry echo in my heart.' He then suddenly awakens to find he has incriminated himself. He commits suicide. Adolfo's innocence is established.

Romani's libretto was so highly regarded that it was set in five subsequent operas: as *Il Sonnambulo* by Luigi Ricci in 1830 and by Carlo Valentini in 1834; as *O Sonambulo* by Luiz Antonio Miró in 1835; and as *Il Fantasma* (*The Ghost*) by Salvatore Agnelli in 1842 and by Giuseppe Persiani in 1843.

Much better known today is Bellini's *La Sonnambula* of 1831, also to a libretto by Romani. This is a work still regularly performed. Count Rodolfo (bass), en route to his castle, takes a room overnight at the village inn. He is warned of a phantom swathed in white that haunts the area at night. The Count, alone in his room, is then disturbed by the young Amina (soprano), sleepwalking and speaking disjointedly. Count Rodolfo refrains from taking advantage of 'this pure and innocent flower' and leaves her asleep in his room. When the villagers arrive to welcome the Count, Amina is discovered in the room and is accused of infidelity to her fiancé Elvino (tenor). But then, in a later scene, before everyone, Amina appears sleepwalking on the roof at the mill-house. All kneel to pray silently for her safety and sigh with relief when she reaches the ground. The villagers now recognize that Amina, 'La Sonnambula', is the dreaded phantom, and that her sleeping presence in the Count's room was innocent. She is restored to her beloved Elvino.

Lady Macbeth's sleepwalking scene from Shakespeare's *Macbeth* has been incorporated largely unchanged into three operas. The French composer Chélard's *Macbeth* to a French libretto by Rouget de Lisle was given at the Paris Opéra in 1827. Despite a brilliant cast, it failed and was withdrawn. A revised version to a German text by Hegel met with more success in Munich in 1828. Nowadays, however, Chélard's opera is rarely performed. Much better known are Verdi's *Macbeth* of 1847 to an Italian libretto by Piave, and Ernest Bloch's *Macbeth* of 1910 to a libretto in French by Edmond Fleg. In Shakespeare and in Verdi the somnambulism is witnessed by a doctor and a lady-in-waiting. Chélard and Bloch omit the doctor.

Lady Macbeth, whose eyes are open 'but their sense is shut', is tormented by her guilt of the murder of King Duncan, reverting over and over again to the stabbing and the torrential bleeding. She tries repeatedly to wash her hands, vainly

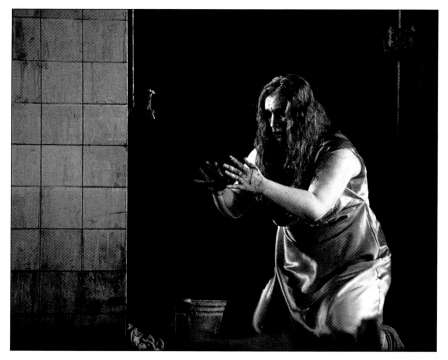

Macbeth (Verdi): The sleepwalking Lady Macbeth (Elisabeth Meister) tries vainly to cleanse her hands of blood. Scottish Opera 2013. Photo: Tommy Ga-Ken Wan.

attempting to cleanse them of supposed bloodstains. This is a vividly dramatic scene in the play and the operas. Parker[1] has praised especially Verdi's expanded formal and harmonic structure and his marvellously inventive orchestration. Kushner[2] points out that Bloch provides the dishevelled Lady Macbeth with vocal pitches more closely associated with speaking, conveying perhaps even greater theatrical effect.

1.	Parker, R., *Grove* III, 113.
2.	Kushner, D. Z., *Grove* III, 114.

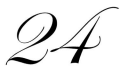

MESMERISM AND HYPNOTISM

I shall deal with these two topics in the same chapter because they are thought by many people to be closely associated. Not rarely, mesmerism and hypnotism are taken as synonymous terms. Both have their practitioners, who often promote their talents publicly. Some of these may well be honestly possessed of valuable remedial skills. Regrettably, however, not a few are fraudulent quacks. There are nevertheless interesting operatic aspects.

MESMERISM

I described Dr Mesmer's career in some detail in my earlier book *Doctors in Opera*; the following is a slightly condensed account. Franz Anton Mesmer was born in 1734. He became much influenced by the activities of a Jesuit priest with the ambiguously suggestive name of Father Hell. Father Hell had, with some apparent success, used magnets for treating the sick. Thus encouraged, Mesmer submitted for his medical graduation at Vienna in 1765 a dissertation concerning the influence of the planets on the human body, in which he proposed that a magnetic fluid pervaded the universe, and affected particularly the nervous system of man and animals. He proceeded to build up a lucrative medical practice involving magnetism which, he claimed, might purposefully divert the course of the supposed magnetic fluid and, if correctly applied, benefit the patient. Not surprisingly, his success seems to have aroused professional jealously, and possibly because of this he moved in 1778 to Paris.

In Paris, Mesmer conducted treatment sessions open to the public at which his patients sat around a special tub or *baquet* clutching iron rods through which the magnetic fluid was supposed to travel. Mesmer approached his patients strangely clad in lilac-coloured silk and carrying a magnet which he waved over them so as to encourage the fluid to flow in the right direction. Quite often at these sessions patients entered a trance or suffered convulsions. Nevertheless, Mesmer also achieved several apparent cures.

King Louis XVI then ordered the French Académie des Sciences to set up a commission to look into the affair. The report of the commission in 1784 rejected Mesmer's magnetic theories, attributing the convulsions and cures that his treatment evoked to the patients' imagination. The commission also pointed out the danger of sexual exploitation of susceptible subjects because of the close rapport often established between doctor and patient in the course of mesmeric treatment. Mesmer died in 1815.

That might have been expected to be the end of mesmerism, but it was not. The French aristocrat Amand-Marie-Jacques de Castanet, Marquis of Puységur (1751–1825) had found that he was easily able to induce a 'mesmeric trance' in a 23-year-old peasant employee, noting a close similarity between the trance-like state and somnambulism (see Chapter 23). Puységur then became a devoted follower of Mesmer and founded an institute for training in 'animal magnetism'. This venture grew rapidly until the French Revolution of 1789, when it was disbanded and Puységur was imprisoned for two years. After the fall of Napoleon in 1815, however, although Mesmer was now dead, Puységur and interest in mesmerism resurfaced.

Independently of Puységur and his followers and initially a sceptic concerning mesmerism, the Scottish surgeon James Braid (1795–1860) observed in 1841 that by getting susceptible persons to focus attention on a fixed object, such as a flickering flame or point of light, he could induce a state of altered consciousness in which the subject showed diminished peripheral awareness with an enhanced tendency to respond to suggestion. Braid was anxious to avoid any association with mesmerism, and his approach became known as hypnotism. He successfully employed this to treat a range of disorders including impaired mobility, headache, various skin complaints, and sensory loss. Such hypnotherapy, as it came to be termed, proceeded to flourish and is nowadays a major pursuit. Mesmerism, in various guises, also continues to thrive and prosper. The aura of vague mysticism surrounding mesmerism evidently has appeal, although few of mesmerism's present-day adherents profess belief in a magnetic fluid pervading the universe.

Dr Mesmer's personal career was neatly bracketed by two of Mozart's operas. In 1768, when Mesmer was at the height of his fame in Vienna, he commissioned the opera *Bastien und Bastienne* by the twelve-year-old Mozart, and the opera was first performed at Mesmer's house in the Landstraße district of Vienna. By 1790 Mesmer had fallen from grace, and Da Ponte, writing the libretto for Mozart's *Così fan Tutte*, was able to make fun of mesmerism. In the opera the maid Despina (soprano) disguises herself as a doctor, and pretends to employ mesmerism so as to treat the fake suicide attempts of Ferrando (tenor) and Guglielmo (baritone). Despina enters brandishing a large magnet ('Doctor Mesmer's stone, first used in Germany and then in France'). Ferrando and Guglielmo each have a suitable convulsion and then recover. The première performance of *Così fan Tutte*, in January 1790, appropriately took place in Vienna, the birthplace of mesmerism.

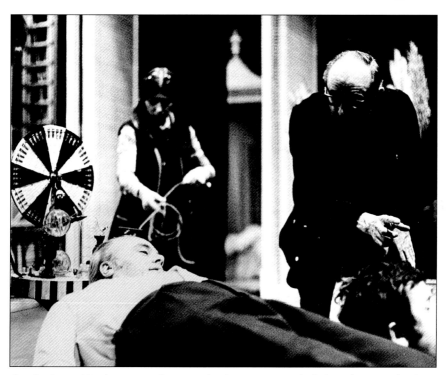

Così fan Tutte: The director Anthony Besch rehearsing Ferrando (Alexander Young), who is feigning illness. Despina (Patricia Hay) here intends evidently to administer mesmerism elaborately via a Wimshurst machine, rather than by the more usual simple magnet. Scottish Opera 1972. Photo: Bob Anderson.

STAGE HYPNOSIS

Whether or not some forms of hypnotism can have genuinely beneficial therapeutic effects, there can be no doubting that stage hypnosis is bogus. Stage hypnosis is performed before an audience for the purpose of entertainment. While there is not overall agreement, most commentators hold that the behaviour seen can be explained by various psychological factors such as disorientation, compliance, peer pressure, and suggestion. Deception by the hypnotist nearly always plays a major part, with various tricks of legerdemain being employed. Preliminary tests, such as asking the audience to clasp their hands and then suggesting they cannot be separated, permit selection of the most compliant subjects. By asking for volunteers to mount the stage, the performer can choose the most extrovert or amenable members of the audience. Participants on stage tend to cooperate because of the social pressures of a situation which has been set up before an expectant audience.

A vividly tragic account of stage hypnotism is given in Thomas Mann's novella *Mario und der Zauberer* (*Mario and the Magician*) of 1929. The story clearly appeals to composers, and has been set as an opera on four occasions: by Stephen Oliver to his own variously Italian or English libretti in 1988; by János Vajda to a Hungarian libretto by Gábor Bókkon in 1989; by Harry Somers to an English libretto by Rod Anderson in 1992; and by Francis Thorne to an English libretto by J. D. McClatchy in 2005. The hypnotist of the story, Cipolla, emphasizes his domination over his subjects by means of a claw-handled whip that he cracks from time to time. Cipolla induces Mario, a quiet young waiter, to join him on stage. Cipolla teases Mario about his love for, and suffering over, a young woman called Silvestra. He then proceeds to convince Mario that he actually sees Silvestra, not Cipolla. Cipolla sings in falsetto, 'Mario, my beloved! Tell me, who am I?' The young man replies, 'Silvestra'. Cipolla then asks, 'Kiss me! Kiss me here – on the lips!' Mario does so. Cipolla suddenly breaks the spell with, 'Ah! my darling! I need breath!' There erupts from the audience loud mocking laughter, and Mario awakens, shocked at what he has just been made to do. Mario starts to run away. Cipolla domineeringly cracks his whip. Mario turns and shoots Cipolla dead. This tale has been seen as an allegorical depiction of fascism, with Cipolla as the self-appointed leader whose demagogic oratory all must obey. With the killing of Cipolla, freedom is regained.

25

INCEST

Incest is not a disease but it is an abnormality.

THE OEDIPUS LEGEND

Numerous operas dealing with the Oedipus legend and derived from the trilogy of plays by the Athenian writer Sophocles were mentioned in the earlier chapter on plague. The gods inflicted that plague on the city of Thebes because of the sins of its king, Oedipus.

The legend tells of a son, Oedipus, born to King Laius and Queen Jocasta of Thebes. Festivities quickly turn to dismay when it is prophesized that the child, born in defiance of the gods, is destined to murder his father and marry his mother. Laius and Jocasta, in a desperate attempt to circumvent the prophecy, order a shepherd to take the infant away and kill him. The shepherd disobeys those instructions, and Oedipus is installed in the palace of King Polybus and Queen Merope of Corinth, whose own infant son has died. Oedipus grows up believing his parents to be Polybus and Merope.

Then, at the age of twenty, Oedipus is told by an oracle of his grim destiny. Convinced that the prediction concerns Polybus and Merope, he leaves Corinth in an attempt to avert his fate. At a crossroads ('where three roads meet') Oedipus encounters, but does not recognise, Laius with two guards. These three wrongly assume that Oedipus, who is unknown to them, is hostile, and attack him. In the ensuing fight Oedipus kills all three. Oedipus proceeds to Thebes, where the population welcomes him and offers him the hand of the recently widowed Jocasta. For some twenty years Oedipus serves as a wise and able king. Thebes prospers and Jocasta bears him healthy children. But then the gods exact retribution. The dreadful truth is revealed. Jocasta commits suicide. Oedipus blinds himself and leaves Thebes as the only sure way of delivering the city from the plague.

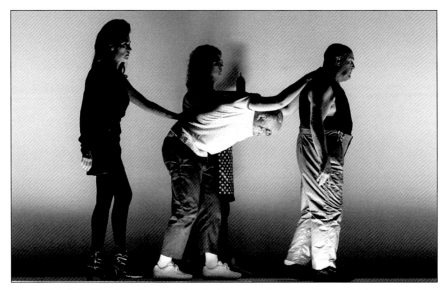

Greek: Eddy (Alex Otterburn), overwhelmed with guilt on learning of his patricide and incest, has blinded himself and is led away by his adoptive parents Dad (Andrew Shore) and Mum (Susan Bullock) together with sister Doreen (Allison Cook, left). Scottish Opera 2017. Photo: Jane Hobson.

OEDIPUS: A LONDON EAST END VARIANT

The opera *Greek* of 1988 by Mark-Anthony Turnage after a play by Steven Berkoff relocates the tale to the East End of London in the late twentieth century. Oedipus becomes Eddy (high baritone) who argues with a café manager (baritone) over croissants, kills him, and marries his wife (mezzo-soprano). But then Eddy's supposed biological parents (baritone and mezzo-soprano) reveal to him that he was adopted ('You're not our son, son'). Eddy has murdered his father and is married to his real mother. The 'plague' is Thatcherite greed and self-interest.

THE PHAEDRA LEGEND

In Greek mythology Phaedra, although married to Theseus, falls in love with Hippolytus, the son of Theseus by another woman. Hippolytus rejects her. In revenge Phaedra claims to Theseus that she has been raped by Hippolytus. Theseus believes Phaedra and curses his son, whose horses are then frightened by a sea monster sent by the god Poseidon. Hippolytus is dragged to his death.

This ancient tale has been incorporated into several operas. Rameau's *Hippolyte et Aricie* of 1733 was to a French libretto by Simon-Joseph Pellegrin. In Act III Phaedra (soprano) declares her love for Hippolytus (haut-contre) but is spurned. Theseus (bass) enters and mistakenly assumes that his son is threatening his wife's virtue. Hippolytus is too honourable to accuse his stepmother by revealing the truth. Theseus prays to Poseidon (bass), who demands the life of Hippolytus.

Then Phaedra, overcome by remorse, kills herself, in her dying moments revealing her guilt to Theseus. The conscience-stricken Theseus is about to throw himself into the sea when Poseidon announces that, through the intervention of Diana (soprano), Hippolytus is alive. However, for too readily accepting his son's guilt, Theseus is condemned never to see him again. This, Rameau's first opera, retains modest popularity and has had several revivals in recent years. Paisiello's *Fedra* of 1788 to a libretto by Salvioni and Pizzetti's *Fedra* of 1915 to a libretto by D'Annunzio also feature the story.

Sylvano Bussotti composed the opera/ballet *Le Racine* of 1980 to his own libretto in French verse after Jean Racine's poem *Phèdre*. The action takes places in a Parisian bar called 'Le Racine' run by a former actress, Madame Phèdre (soprano), who recites Racine's verses. Musical accompaniment is provided just by piano, reflecting the piano-bar setting. The initial incestuous relationship is between Madame Phèdre and Hippolyte, a dancer. However, the author Racine (bass) also takes part in the action. As father-figure to the characters, he commits incest with Hippolyte. Bussotti later reworked *Le Racine* as a three-act lyric tragedy, *Fedre*, with full orchestra, first given in Rome in 1988.

The opera *Phaedra* of 2007 by Hans Werner Henze is to a German-language libretto by Christian Lehnert. Act I follows the ancient tale closely, with the guilty Phaedra, sung by a mezzo-soprano, at the end killing herself in remorse after the death of Hippolytus (tenor). Act II is derived from a mythological account attributed to Ovid. Hippolytus is restored to life by Artemis, the latter in the opera an epicene character sung by a countertenor. The revived Hippolytus is brought to Nemi, near Henze's home in Italy, and the location of the ancient cult of Virbius. Action becomes increasingly abstract and nebulous. The opera dissolves away into inconclusive transcendence.

WAGNERIAN INCEST

There is an interesting pattern of incest at the centre of Wagner's great operatic tetralogy *Der Ring des Nibelungen*. In the second opera, *Die Walküre*, Siegmund (heldentenor) and Sieglinde (soprano) are the twin children of Wotan (bass-baritone) by an anonymous mother. They have long been separated. Sieglinde has been married for several years to Hunding (bass), but that union has thus far been sterile. Seeking shelter from a storm, Siegmund finds the dwelling of Hunding and Sieglinde and is taken in. Siegmund and Sieglinde recognise each other and immediately fall in love. This is far more than sibling endearment; it is passionate sexual desire. Sieglinde drugs Hunding. By the end of Act I Sieglinde, in contradistinction to her barren years with Hunding, is pregnant by her twin brother Siegmund. Sieglinde's delirium of early pregnancy is discussed in the following chapter.

The child of their union is Siegfried (heldentenor). In the third opera of the tetralogy, entitled *Siegfried*, that hero discovers the sleeping Brünnhilde (soprano) at a mountain-top fastness protected by a ring of fire. Siegfried fearlessly penetrates the flames, awakens Brünnhilde with a kiss, and takes her as his bride. Brünnhilde is the daughter of Wotan and Erda (contralto), and is hence half-sister to Siegmund and Sieglinde, both of whom are now dead. Siegfried has therefore married his aunt. That pair die without issue.

In the nineteenth century, when *Der Ring* first appeared (Wagner published the text several years before the entire tetralogy was first staged in 1876), many people were shocked by these incestuous affairs. The union between Siegmund and Sieglinde was widely considered to be particularly offensive. Twenty-first-century audiences are usually more tolerant. Incest, whether or not it is found to be disturbing by some of the audience, does not however noticeably upset the characters in Wagner's *Der Ring* and hence does not influence the development of the drama.

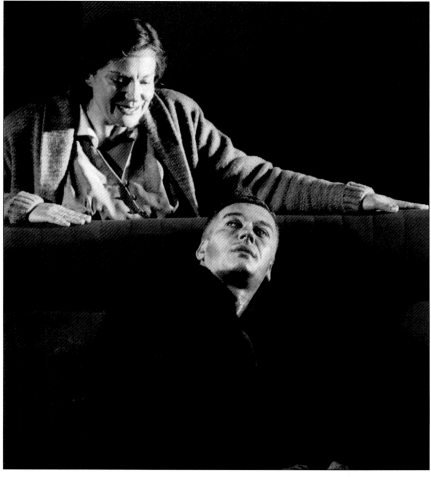

Die Walküre: The incestuous twins Sieglinde (Ursula Füri-Bernhard) and Siegmund (Jan Kyhle). Scottish Opera 2001. Photo: Bill Cooper.

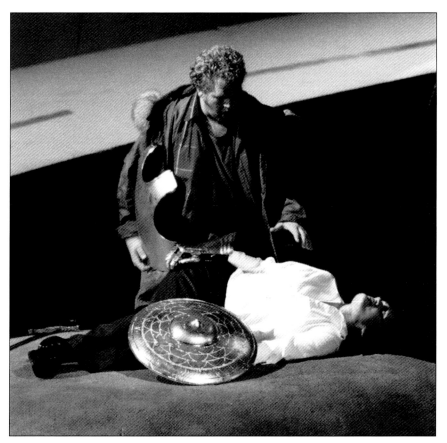

Siegfried: Siegfried (Graham Sanders) about to waken his aunt Brünnhilde (Elizabeth Byrne) and take her as his bride. Scottish Opera 2002. Photo: Bill Cooper.

PARISIAN INCEST

The characters in Wagner's *Der Ring* display an insouciant attitude towards incest. Circumstances are very different in the French composer Méhul's *Mélidore et Phrosine* of 1794, to a libretto by Arnault. Here the problem of incest is taken much more seriously and is central to the course of events.

Phrosine (soprano) loves, and hopes to marry, Mélidore (haute-contre), although her brother Aimar (baritone) wishes her to wed someone of higher rank. When she attempts to enlist the support of her other brother Jules (tenor), she is shocked to discover that Jules loves her incestuously. When Phrosine persists in her love for Mélidore, Jules, in a jealous rage, tries to murder her. She is saved by Mélidore. Jules then realizes the enormity of his crime, begs his sister's forgiveness, and forswears his incestuous love. All rejoice at the happy outcome. However, the dramatic theme of incest was unacceptable to many of the Parisian audience of the day, and cut short the opera's run at the Opéra-Comique.

INCEST LEADING TO MURDER

Kurt Weill's opera *Der Protagonist* of 1926 was to a libretto by Georg Kaiser. The Protagonist (tenor), leader of a troupe of strolling players, has an incestuous relationship with his sister Catherine (soprano). Then Catherine falls in love with a young gentleman (baritone) and is obliged to confess this to her incredulous brother. Later, from the street, the Protagonist catches sight of Catherine rehearsing a scene in which she has to caress extravagantly an elderly gentleman. The Protagonist mistakes this for real life, rushes in, and in a jealous rage stabs his sister to death.

INCEST TOGETHER WITH MULTIPLE DISEASES

Edgar Allen Poe's tale of grotesque sinister horror, *The Fall of the House of Usher*, dating from 1839, has been set as an opera on at least four occasions. Claude Debussy's *La Chute de la Maison Usher* to his own French libretto remained unfinished at his death in 1918. Sitsky's *The Fall of the House of Usher* of 1965 was to an English libretto by Gwen Harwood. Glass's *The Fall of the House of Usher* of 1988 also had English text, by Arthur Yorinks. Gordon Getty's *Usher House* of 2014 was to his own English libretto.

Poe's story and the operas derived from it are remarkable for the wide range of medical disorders they contain. Roderick Usher and his twin sister Madeline are both of them unmarried and childless. They are the last of their genealogical line, the House of Usher. The pair of them live in their gloomy crumbling castle, also termed the House of Usher. Roderick has severe mental depression plus agoraphobia, the latter a psychological dread of leaving his dwelling. He suffers also from a morbid hyperacuity of all five senses; he can bear hardly anything to touch his skin; he shuns the light; he can tolerate the sounds only of soft-stringed instruments such as the guitar; the scents of flowers are unbearable to him; and he can endure only the most insipid food. Madeline Usher is wasting away with anorexia nervosa, a condition in which the patient refuses to eat. Madeline also has attacks of catalepsy, a disease marked by the sudden arrest of all movements and the prolonged maintenance of distorted physical postures. From time to time, and simultaneous with her episodes of catalepsy, Madeline enters a trance-like mental state. The wording of Poe's tale strongly suggests, but does not state explicitly, that there had once been an incestuous relationship between Roderick and Madeline. Their present torpor, however, precludes sexual activity.

Then Madeline is found to be unrousable and is pronounced dead. Her body is conveyed to a distant room of the castle, her coffin lid is screwed down, and the door firmly secured. Over the next week Roderick becomes more and more distracted. A wild storm erupts one night. A distant, but increasingly loud, knocking obtrudes. Roderick announces that he has heard this frightening noise several times on recent nights, and he fears that it may come from the coffin of his sister, whom he now dreads has been entombed while still alive. A horrific medical error has indeed been made; one of Madeline's cataleptic trances has been mistaken for her death. There is an abrupt rasping crash as of the rending of the wooden lid of her coffin; there can be heard the grating of the hinges of the door of her prison; and then suddenly, at the threshold, there stands the enshrouded figure of Madeline in bloodstained white robes. She reels for a moment, then with a horrible moan falls upon her brother, and in her final death throes carries him, now also a corpse, to the floor. Their incestuous love has been carried through to death.

The storm increases in its intensity. A great split appears in the castle wall. Then the whole building collapses into the moat. The House of Usher, the castle and the genealogical line, both have fallen, for ever.

26

PREGNANCY, CHILDBIRTH, AND MISCARRIAGE

Pregnancy and childbirth are regular physiological events which readily incur complications and are therefore, for those involved, nearly always of paramount concern or even anxiety. Opera is drama; hence, when childbirth is presented in opera, abnormalities are to be expected and disquiet is prevalent. Inevitably, maternal unease is likely to be greatest with the first pregnancy and delivery. Operatic childbirth nearly always involves the first pregnancy.

DELIRIUM OF EARLY PREGNANCY

Early pregnancy, especially a first pregnancy, can feature swings of mood and occasionally frank delirium. Sieglinde displays this in Act II scene 3 of Wagner's *Die Walküre.* As was described in the previous chapter, Sieglinde has just been impregnated by her twin brother Siegmund, and the guilty pair are now fleeing from her irate husband Hunding. Sieglinde is raving:

> Away! Away!
> Flee from one who's defiled!
> ... this body is dead:
> flee from the corpse ...
> May the wind waft her away
> ... Forsake the accursed creature,
> let her flee far away!
> Depraved am I
> and devoid of all worth![1]

This is the nearest Wagner came to writing a mad scene.

PARTURITION (LABOUR)

Explicitly and virtually exclusively obstetric is David Bruce's chamber opera *Push!* of 2006, to a libretto by Anna Reynolds. It depicts a series of women having a baby.

Nimmy (soprano) has detailed requests concerning her delivery: 'I'd really like to NOT have, like, drugs? I don't wanna lie down, so if I do, get me up! We're gonna so have some incense and patchouli oil and stuff in the room if that's kool. Can we use the birthing pool? And does my bloke need to bring his trunks? Please don't shave my pubes!!! Unless you have to of course for the baby's sake, it really icks me even to THINK about it.'

Cara (soprano) has multiple partners, which obviously incurs social problems: 'Under no circumstances should any of my husbands be allowed into the delivery room. I do not, repeat not, want to be offered an epidural. Just say NO. I would like my acupuncturist to be at the birth but if she's busy with Madonna or Kylie, then her assistant will do. I do not intend to breastfeed – so last decade – so please have a bottle ready.'

Maddy (soprano) is in prison and is handcuffed to the hospital bed when giving birth. Her baby is to be adopted: 'The prisoner would not like any drugs during the birth, no matter how bad the pain gets. The prisoner would prefer not to see the child when it is born but to hand it over straight away. The prisoner would not like music, incense or any soothing nonsense.'

Mary (soprano) has been impregnated by *in vitro* fertilisation (IVF), which has gone slightly wrong and she is now expecting quintuplets. 'I'd like to float away

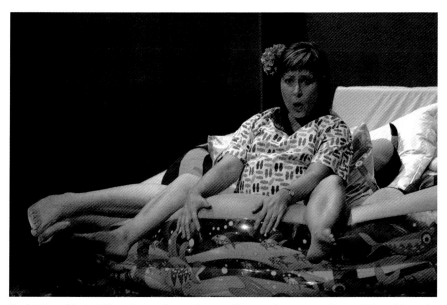

Push!: Cara (Rachel Hynes), together with one of her sundry partners (James Edwards), in the birthing pool. Tête à Tête 2006. Photo: Suzanne Jansen.

on a combination of gas, air and dreamy dreams please. I'd like my husband to be at my side, although due to an unfortunate absence ever since the conception, he won't be here. However, if he does appear, please show him in! I understand women in labour can be irrational – so please ignore me when I begin shouting and cursing, I'm only bloody human after all. Please put all my babies onto my tummy as soon as they are born – I'm so fat there will probably be room.'

Angela is a mezzo-soprano. Her baby has died in the womb. She knows he will be stillborn. Her requests are harrowing: 'I would like someone to take photographs of my baby as he is born. I know this will be unbearably hard. I am so sorry that I have to ask this. I need to see what he looked like you see ... It's all I will have. If I cry, don't try to comfort me. Just let me be. After the birth, please let me have some time alone with the body. I have brought some clothes. They are special. Please let me dress him.'

And then there is the Cleaner (soprano), who is pregnant by the hospital caretaker (baritone). She is asked about her birth plan: 'A birth plan? Yes, I plan to give birth. Thank you. Oh. I see. A plan for how. I would like everything possible to be done for the safety of my baby. I never thought I would have one, you see. I don't want any fuss. I'm only having a baby. People do it all the time.'

In two operas, labour is required to proceed in unusually disturbing surroundings. Kurt Weill's *Street Scene* of 1947 is to a libretto by Elmer Rice after his own play. Dr Wilson (spoken) delivers Mrs Buchanan of her baby in a New York heatwave to the accompaniment, in an adjoining apartment, of the murder of Anna Maurrant (soprano) and her lover Steve Sankey (spoken) by the jealous husband Frank Maurrant (bass-baritone).

Jonathan Dove's *Flight* of 1998 was composed to a text by April De Angelis. The Minskwoman (mezzo-soprano) successfully gives birth in a crowded airport

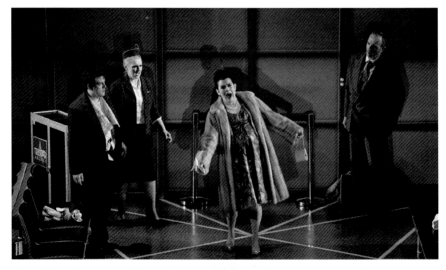

Flight: The Minskwoman (Victoria Simmonds) goes into labour in the airport departure lounge. Also present are the Steward (Jonathan McGovern), Stewardess (Sioned Gwen Davies), and Minskman (Stephen Gadd). Scottish Opera 2018. Photo: James Glossop.

departure lounge despite the absence of professional care. This is not a location many women would favour for their first, or indeed any, confinement, although whether the word confinement is appropriate to these circumstances could be questioned.

POSTPARTUM INFECTION (CHILDBED FEVER; PUERPERAL SEPSIS)

Postpartum sepsis is a bacterial infection of the female reproductive tract following childbirth or miscarriage. It occurs usually after the first 24 hours and within the first ten days following delivery, the most common involvement being of the uterus and surrounding tissues. Causation was clarified with the discovery of bacteria and the recognition of bacterial infection in the late nineteenth century. The twentieth century development of antibiotics provided effective therapy. Long before these insights there had been strong suspicions that imperfect hygiene of attendant doctors was responsible, one of the earliest warnings being uttered in 1795 by the Scottish obstetrician Alexander Gordon.

Ignaz Semmelweis (1818–65) was a Hungarian-born physician of German descent working in the Vienna General Hospital. He observed in 1847 that the incidence of puerperal infection was much higher in the First Maternity Clinic, staffed by doctors, than in the Second Clinic, staffed by midwives. Doctors routinely went from the post-mortem room and performing autopsies to the

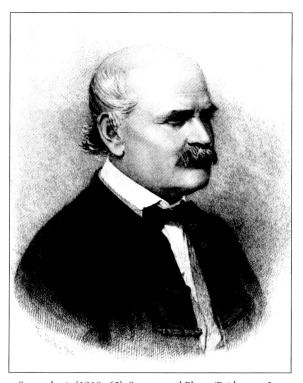

Ignaz Semmelweis (1818–65). Spaarnestad Photo/Bridgeman Images.

maternity clinic without washing their hands. Semmelweis concluded that the doctors were thus in some way transmitting the disease from cadavers to mothers. Although he could at that time provide no scientific explanation, Semmelweis published his findings, with the recommendation that doctors should wash their hands thoroughly before attending the maternity clinic. The medical profession was outraged. It was unacceptable that earnest, dedicated doctors should be seen as the immediate cause of a deadly disease. The ideas of Semmelweis were mocked and ridiculed, he was dismissed from his post, became mentally deranged, and was admitted to an asylum where he died aged just 47. Posthumously Semmelweis was thoroughly vindicated by Pasteur's confirmation of the germ theory of disease and the success of Lister's antiseptic techniques.

Semmelweis is a theatrical opera/song cycle composed by Raymond J. Lustig to a libretto by Matthew Doherty. It had its premiere staging in Budapest in September 2018, two hundred years after the birth of Semmelweis. A New York concert performance had been given a year earlier. The work, in one act, runs for some 75 minutes, with movement, staging, lighting, back-projection and voiceover conveying the narrative. The title role is sung by a bass-baritone, with a female chorus representing variously patients, mothers, midwives, and nurses. Four instrumentalists (piano/organ, percussion, strings) are supplemented by various onstage instruments played by members of the chorus. The action includes an autopsy and a delivery.

This clearly very powerfully dramatic work was well received.

MATERNAL DEATH

Maternal deaths in opera occur variously on and off the stage; there follow accounts of three of each variety.

Claude Debussy composed his opera *Pelléas et Mélisande* of 1902 to a libretto edited by himself from the play of that name by the Belgian writer Maeterlinck. In the final act, Mélisande (soprano), the wife of Golaud (baritone), has just given birth to a healthy daughter. In performance, delivery has usually occurred before the rise of the curtain, but an occasional director has the birth take place on the open stage. Mélisande is clearly very unwell. This could be a consequence not of problems at parturition, but of earlier beatings she has been given by her jealous husband. The onset is too early for puerperal sepsis. The attending Doctor (bass) reassures Golaud that the blows Mélisande received were light and unlikely to cause serious harm. Nevertheless, Mélisande dies. Whether this is a result of Golaud's assaults, or of blood loss at or following delivery, is left unclear.

The chamber opera *The Juniper Tree* of 1985 by Philip Glass and Robert Moran is to a libretto by Arthur Yorinks. It is possibly Glass's most popular opera. The Mother (soprano) wishes intensely for a child, becomes pregnant, but dies giving birth to the Son (soprano). The Father (baritone) remarries and provides the Son with a half-sister, the Daughter (soprano). The Stepmother (mezzo-

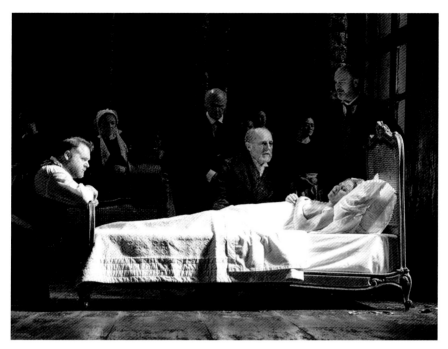

Pelléas et Mélisande: Mélisande (Carolyn Sampson) has given birth to a daughter but is dying. Around her bed are (left to right) her husband Golaud (Roland Wood), Golaud's grandfather Arkel (Alistair Miles) and the Doctor (Jonathan May). Scottish Opera 2017. Photo: Richard Campbell.

soprano) becomes pathologically jealous of the Son, leading to dramatic events of extreme complexity, albeit all turns out well in the end.

A most spectacularly complicated on-stage maternal death is seen in Judith Weir's *A Night at the Chinese Opera* of 1987, composed to her own libretto. The heavily pregnant Mrs Chao (soprano) has the misfortune of observing her husband (tenor) stabbing himself to death, whereupon she is obliged unaided to drag his body off stage. There are compelling practical reasons why she has to do this. This passage of the opera is a play within the overall drama, and is being enacted by just three singers – soprano, mezzo-soprano, and tenor – who must take multiple roles. The body has to be removed so that the tenor can return to play the part of the doctor. So Mrs Chao removes the corpse, re-enters, and is successfully delivered of a son. But as the tenor, who has now reappeared as her physician Dr Ch'êng Ying, is prescribing herbal medicines for her to take after her confinement, she unaccountably strangles herself. The doctor is left holding the baby.

In three other operas the audience learns of a mother's death when giving birth. Here the events are narrated, not presented on stage. Yet all three bear crucially on the subsequent drama.

In Wagner's *Siegfried* of 1876 the dwarf Mime (tenor) tells the young Siegfried (heldentenor) how he discovered Siegfried's stricken mother Sieglinde giving

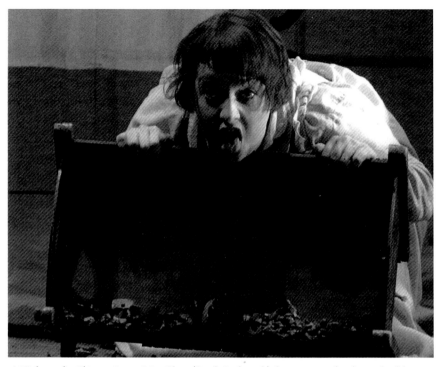

A Night at the Chinese Opera: Mrs Chao (Sarah Redgwick), having given birth to a healthy son, unaccountably strangles herself. Scottish Opera 2008. Photo: Richard Campbell.

birth, and how she died despite Mime's ministrations. Siegfried comes to believe for a time that all mothers die at delivery. Mime raises Siegfried as if he were his own child, intending to use him as a means of gaining possession of the all-powerful Ring. But Siegfried perceives Mime's dissembling manipulations and in exasperation kills him.

Poulenc's *Dialogues des Carmélites* was composed in 1957 to his own libretto after a play by Georges Bernanos. Blanche de la Force (soprano) has learnt that her mother died giving birth to her. This knowledge has evidently disturbed her mentally, causing her to be constantly anxious and readily frightened. She becomes a nun at a Carmelite convent, hoping that this will provide a protective refuge and calm her fears.

Sally Beamish's opera *Monster* of 2002 to a libretto by Janice Galloway tells of the events leading up to Mary Shelley's authorship of her novel *Frankenstein: The Modern Prometheus*, published in 1818. Mary Shelley's mother, Mary Wollstonecraft, had died giving her birth. Mary Wollstonecraft seems to have been a rather domineering person, inclined to proffer peremptory instructions to all and sundry. It might be thought that her death would have protected the daughter from such harassment, but in the opera that turns out not to be so. Composer and librettist contrived to insert the dead mother into the opera, casting her as a contralto, and having her spirit step out of her portrait from time to time to deliver harangues.

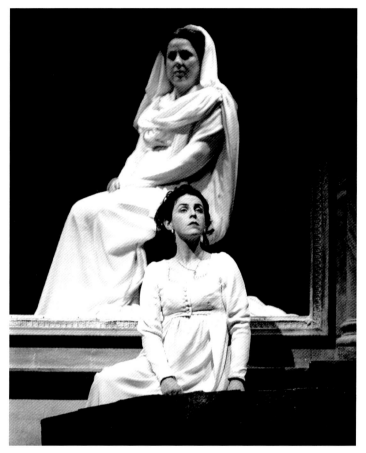

Mary Wollstonecraft (Claire Shearer) about to step out of her portrait to harangue her daughter Mary Shelley (Gail Pearson). Scottish Opera 2002. Photo: Bill Cooper.

MISCARRIAGE

Not all operatic pregnancies go to their full term. A spectacular miscarriage occurs in Samuel Barber's *Vanessa* of 1958, composed to a libretto by Gian-Carlo Menotti. The action is set in 1905 at Vanessa's opulent country house, vaguely stated to be 'somewhere in Northern Europe'. Nevertheless, wherever in Northern Europe it is, the characters speak English, which narrows the possibilities considerably. Those possibilities are restricted even further by the staging of a lively Hogmanay party. At that party the bibulous Doctor (bass-baritone) is to announce the engagement between Vanessa (soprano) and Anatol (tenor). Unknown to them all, however, Vanessa's niece, Erika (mezzo-soprano) is pregnant as a result of an earlier encounter with Anatol. As the intoxicated Doctor begins his speech, Erika suddenly rushes out into the snowy night, crying 'His child! ... must not be born!' She attempts suicide by jumping into a ravine. This results in miscarriage but not her death. Although Vanessa suspects what has happened, the full truth is kept from her. The marriage goes ahead.

The Polish composer Penderecki's opera *The Devils of Loudon* of 1969 is based on a true story dating from the 1630s which was recounted in detail in a book by Aldous Huxley.[2] The tale was then dramatised by John Whiting and it is from Whiting's play that Penderecki derived his libretto. A central figure is the priest, Father Urbain Grandier, a baritone in the opera; handsome, personable, articulate, a compelling preacher, and a womaniser. Grandier is invited by Sister Jeanne (soprano), Prioress of St Ursula's Convent, to be their Director and Confessor to the order, an invitation which he regretfully declines. But very soon after this, Sister Jeanne begins to experience sexual fantasies based on Grandier, who she comes to believe has sent various devils as emissaries to possess her carnally. Sexual hysteria spreads rapidly from the Prioress through the convent, with several other Ursuline sisters claiming to have engaged in sexual acts with demons sent especially by Grandier for that purpose. Grandier is arrested, tried, found guilty of sorcery, and burnt at the stake.

Although Penderecki's opera ends at that point, the real-life historical events continued in a most interesting fashion and merit retelling. According to the Prioress, Isacaaron, the devil of concupiscence, appeared, took advantage of her, and made her pregnant. Perhaps fortunately, the pregnancy miscarried, that miscarriage being, by her account, spontaneous.

1. Translation by Stewart Spencer, in *Wagner's Ring of the Nibelung: A Companion*, edited by Spencer, S. and Millington, B., Thames & Hudson, London, 1993, 157.

2. Huxley, A., *The Devils of Loudun*, Chatto & Windus, London, 1952.

27

HERBAL MEDICINE

TRISTAN AND ISOLDE

A major duty of a medieval matriarch was to prepare and maintain a herbal pharmacopoeia. These medicines would be used to treat illnesses, heal wounds, act as sedatives or aphrodisiacs, and so forth. Isolde's mother, who was just such a matriarch, had included a selection of drugs in Isolde's trousseau when Isolde departed from Ireland to be married to the Cornish King Marke. These had been entrusted to the care of Isolde's lady-in-waiting, Brangäne. One of the drugs was an aphrodisiac intended for the ageing King Marke. This is explicit in the secular oratorio by the Swiss composer Frank Martin, *Le Vin Herbé*, dating from 1941. Martin took as his libretto the text of the nineteenth-century French writer Joseph Bédier, and he set Bédier's words almost unchanged. This is the English translation at the relevant passage:

> When the time came to deliver Isolde to the Knights of Cornwall, her mother gathered herbs, flowers and roots, and mixed them with wine and made a potent drink … she poured this into a goblet and said to Brangäne: 'Take this wine goblet … as the wedding night approaches and just before the newlyweds are left alone … pour this wine into a cup and offer it to them, seeing that they both, King Marke and Queen Isolde, drain it together.'

The supposed aphrodisiac would almost certainly include extracts of plants of the solanacae (belladonna) family. One of Wagner's principal sources for his *Tristan und Isolde*, Gottfried von Strassburg,[1] was well aware of the employment of belladonna extracts in this context. There are known to be two principal active chemicals in extracts from solanaceae plants – the alkaloids atropine and hyoscine. Both are in wide use in medicine today and their properties are clearly understood and defined. They are anticholinergic, meaning that they antagonise the effects of the activator acetylcholine on the autonomic (unconscious) nervous system.

With progressively increasing doses there will be dry mouth; widening of the pupils of the eye with marked visual disturbance and intolerance of light, although the ability to see in the dark will be enhanced; rapid heart rate; palpitations; skin flushing; hallucinations; delirium; coma; and death following big doses. The effects on the eye are emphasized because although they occur at low doses they are often very prolonged, not rarely lasting several days. The term 'belladonna' – 'beautiful woman' – derives from the property of pupil widening, which was once supposed to make a woman more attractive. Whether solanaceae extracts are genuinely aphrodisiac is more questionable, but in this field suggestion can be very powerful, especially when combined with delirium and hallucinations.

Wagner's opera of 1865 was to his own text. In Act I Tristan (tenor) and Isolde (soprano) realise that they are passionately in love. Yet their situation is seemingly impossible to resolve, as Tristan is the envoy sent to Ireland to escort Isolde by ship to Cornwall and there wed his uncle King Marke (bass). They decide on double suicide. Isolde orders Brangäne (mezzo-soprano) to bring them a deadly poison. But Brangäne panics and proffers instead the supposed aphrodisiac. Any aphrodisiac properties of their drink are in the circumstances superfluous. But as Gunther Weitz emphasized in a very perceptive article,[2] both Tristan and Isolde immediately display marked features of solanaceae ingestion. According to Wagner's stage directions, they are seized with trembling, they clutch convulsively at their hearts, they raise their hands to their heads, their eyes seek out each other, but are cast down in confusion. All these features can be seen as corresponding to solanaceae intoxication, by indicating fast heart rate, palpitations, facial flushing, and blurred vision. The two then embrace, wildly declare their love for each other, and are oblivious to their surroundings. Brangäne becomes very alarmed. The ship docks. Tristan is told King Marke is approaching: 'Who? What King?' Isolde also is utterly confused: 'Why are they calling out? ... Am I alive? ... Where am I? ... What was in that drink?' Isolde falls unconscious. Act I ends with both Tristan and Isolde thus displaying remarkably faithful symptoms and signs of solanaceae (belladonna) toxicity.

Wagner does not make clear how long elapses from the end of Act I to the beginning of Act II, but it appears to be at most a day or so. That brief interval would be important in that effects of solanaceae on the eyes could readily persist over that time. Those long-lasting features would be widening of the pupils of the eyes, resulting in failure of accommodation and therefore blurring of vision, plus intolerance of light. Conversely, ability to see in the dark would be enhanced.

King Marke and his court proceed on a nocturnal hunting expedition. Tristan slips away and joins Isolde in an illicit tryst. The two ardently declare their love. Their mutual exclamations are littered with references to their intolerance of light, their dislike of daylight, their inability to see clearly in bright light, their conversely enhanced nocturnal vision, and hence their preference for night.

Their amorous exchanges include such assertions as, 'Oh, now we are dedicated to Night ... spiteful Day is mocked by those to whom Night has granted sight ...

fleeting flashes of light no longer dazzle us ... etc.'. Many commentators take this to be just poetic symbolism. Notwithstanding, Weitz sees it as distinct evidence of the pharmacological action of solanaceae alkaloids.

The two lovers are then surprised by the return and sudden irruption of King Marke with his courtiers, including the knight Melot (tenor). Many of the retinue are carrying torches. Moreover, it is dawn. Illumination from both of those sources would be unwelcome to persons under the influence of solanaceae alkaloids, so it is hardly anomalous that Tristan, again complaining about the light, covers Isolde, including her face, with his cloak and stares, we are told, sightlessly at the others. After a long, sad aria from King Marke, there is a sudden strange ending to Act II. Tristan rushes upon Melot to attack him: 'Defend yourself Melot!' Tristan

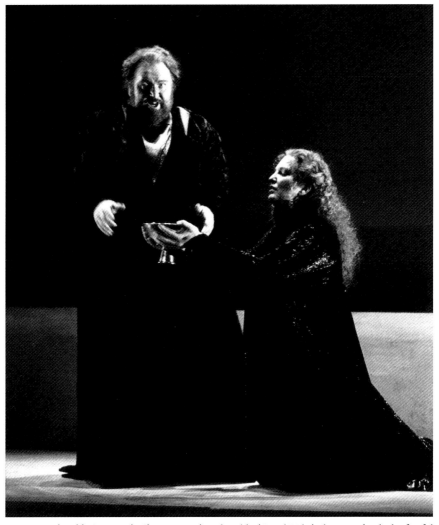

Tristan und Isolde: Tristan (Jeffrey Lawton) and Isolde (Carol Yahr) about to drink the fateful potion. Scottish Opera 1994. Photo: Clive Barda.

then unaccountably lowers his sword and allows Melot to wound him. Many see this as Tristan deliberately seeking death. But it could be that Tristan, still under the influence of solanaceae, cannot see properly, and is in no condition to fight.

Wagner was not a pharmacologist, and he could hardly have been expected to be familiar with the detailed actions of atropine and hyoscine. But he could have read descriptive accounts of the effects of solanaceae extracts. It has to be conceded, however, that the proposals of Weitz have not been widely accepted. But I find them to be persuasively perceptive.

SIEGFRIED'S AMNESIA

Weitz and I[3] went on to try to explain Siegfried's loss of memory in Wagner's *Götterdämmerung* of 1876, the fourth opera of his great tetralogy, *Der Ring des Nibelungen*. Siegfried (tenor) takes his leave of his wife Brünnhilde (soprano) in order, so he says, to seek new adventures. He leaves her apparently secure at her mountain-top fastness, surrounded by a protective circle of fire and in possession of the supposedly all-powerful golden Ring. Siegfried arrives at the Hall of the Gibichungs and is welcomed by Gunther (baritone) and Gutrune (soprano), unmarried brother and sister, and by their half-brother Hagen (bass). Hagen is the son of Alberich, who is determined if possible to regain the Ring. Hagen directs Gutrune to prepare a drink for Siegfried. Siegfried swallows this, and at once apparently forgets his recent past. He declares ardent love for Gutrune, whom he met only a few minutes earlier, and proposes marriage. He then volunteers to bring Brünnhilde down from her mountain refuge to be the bride of Gunther. With the aid of a magic helmet, the Tarnhelm, which enables him to change shape at will, and which can also provide instantaneous transportation, Siegfried does this. In the guise of Gunther he penetrates the circle of fire, wrests the Ring from Brünnhilde's finger, and returns with her to the Gibichung Hall, where he hands her over to Gunther. Gunther weds Brünnhilde and Siegfried weds Gutrune. Siegfried, at least for the time being, retains the Ring.

Then the following day, on a hunting expedition, Hagen gives Siegfried a drink which is an antidote to the first. Siegfried recovers his memory and blurts out the truth that he had once been married to Brünnhilde. Hagen accuses him of treachery and kills him by stabbing him in the back, Siegfried's one vulnerable place. Hagen tries but fails to detach the Ring from the dead Siegfried's finger.

After much debate, Weitz and I decided that the initial welcoming drink which caused Siegfried to lose his recent memory probably contained solanaceae extract. If so, any externally evident effects are much less marked than those seen in *Tristan und Isolde*. Hagen does remark on Siegfried's reddened cheeks, which might suggest a solanaceae-induced flush. The sudden infatuation with Gutrune could indicate sexual stimulation. But quite unlike Tristan and Isolde, Siegfried is never confused, stupefied, hallucinated, or disorientated, and he has no disturbance of vision. If Siegfried's first drink did contain anticholinergic plant extracts, the second, which restored his memory, would have comprised probably a direct antidote. According to this notion the second drink could have contained physostigmine extracted from the calabar bean, or muscarine obtained from fly agaric. Physostigmine or muscarine would overcome the blocking actions of atropine and hyoscine on the autonomic nervous system, and hence would return Siegfried to normal (or at any rate to as nearly normal as someone such as Siegfried could be expected to become).

Weitz and I thus agreed on the likely contents of the two fateful drinks. However, we disagreed on our conclusions. Weitz saw Siegfried as a naive, innocent hero, whose amnesia was genuinely induced by solanaceae extract, and whose actions thereafter were largely unwitting. I more cynically considered that the initial dose was insufficient to produce substantial effects; that Siegfried had tired of Brünnhilde's charms; that he was ready to fall for Gutrune (or any suitable lass) and simulated his loss of memory. We invited readers to decide for themselves on these alternatives. I have to concede that so far many more have agreed with Weitz than with me.

There is one further aspect, which may help some readers. Oysters are sometimes recommended as an alternative aphrodisiac; indeed, one Glasgow fishmonger has a notice outside his shop claiming that his oysters are superior to Viagra.[4] Presumably neither Hagen nor Isolde's mother had ready access to oysters.

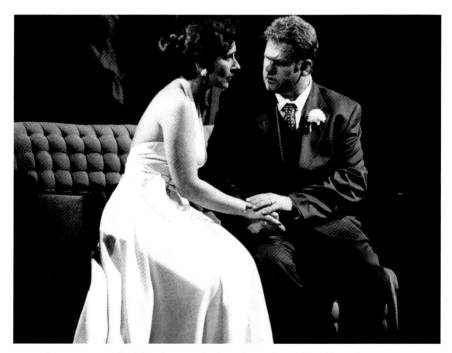

Götterdämmerung: Siegfried (Graham Sanders), suffering drug-induced loss of memory, proposes bigamous marriage to Gutrune (Elaine McKrill). Scottish Opera 2003. Photo: Bill Cooper.

A HERB TO CURE ADULTEROUS LOVE

A herb with very different properties is sought in two operas based on the same true story concerning the assassination of King Gustavus III of Sweden. These are Auber's *Gustave III* or *Le Bal Masqué* of 1833 to a French libretto by Scribe, and Verdi's *Un Ballo in Maschera* of 1859 to an Italian libretto by Somma adapted from Scribe. Strict censorship required Verdi and Somma to change the names of the characters and the country of the action; for the sake of clarity I have kept here the original names and location.

Amélie/Amelia (soprano), wife of Count Ankarström (bass or baritone), is conducting an illicit liaison with the Swedish King Gustavus (tenor). She has been advised to visit the place of the gallows at midnight, where she may obtain a herb ('una magica erba') which will cure her adulterous love.[5] One might suppose that it would be easier to find a rare plant in daylight, but of course midnight is operatically more dramatic. The identity of the herb remains obscure. The traditional gallows plant is mandrake, which was once believed to derive from semen dripping from hanged criminals. But mandrake, described by Banquo in Shakespeare's *Macbeth* as 'the insane root that takes the reason prisoner', is an unlikely candidate for curing adultery. In any event, the King suddenly arrives on the scene and all thought of sexual rectitude is abandoned. Amelia's illicit affair continues and is discovered by her husband, who then murders the King.

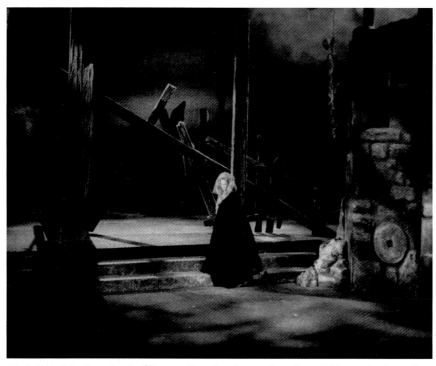

Un Ballo in Maschera: Amelia (Cristina Deutekom) visits the gallows field at midnight, seeking a herb to assuage her adulterous love for the King. Scottish Opera 1975. Photo: Eric Thorburn.

ROMEO AND JULIET

The story of Romeo and Juliet is probably the most popular of all with opera composers and has been set on very many occasions. Although best known from Shakespeare's play, it originated earlier, probably in an Italian romance by Matteo Bandello. The two most prominent survivors into the present-day operatic repertoire are Gounod's *Roméo et Juliette* of 1867 to a libretto by Barbier and Carré and Bellini's *I Capuleti e i Montecchi* of 1830 to a libretto by Romani. Barbier and Carré based their libretto for Gounod on Shakespeare. However, Romani derived his text for Bellini not via Shakespeare but from an 1818 play by Luigi Scevola, itself an adaptation of a previous account. The composer Hector Berlioz was an admirer of Shakespeare and of the Shakespearean actress Harriet Smithson, whom he later married. When Berlioz saw a performance in Paris of the Bellini version, he much lamented the omission of several Shakespearean characters and events.[6]

In both operas a powerful herbal medicine is administered to Juliet, in Gounod's by the herbalist Friar Laurence (bass), in Bellini's by Doctor Lorenzo (tenor or bass). This drug, taken by mouth, has a prolonged general anaesthetic action – 'two and forty hours' according to Friar Laurence. It also induces features of hibernation, with breathing and heartbeat being almost, if not wholly, imperceptible. Unfortunately, when Juliet awakes after the forty-two hours are up, she finds that Romeo, who had supposed her dead, has committed suicide, and his body lies beside her. Juliet also kills herself.

HERBAL VETERINARY MEDICINE

A rare operatic appearance of a veterinary practitioner is made in Darius Milhaud's *Les Malheurs d'Orphée* (*The Misfortunes of Orpheus*). This work, to a libretto by Armand Lunel, dates from 1926. Orpheus (baritone) employs herbal remedies to treat sick animals. He is remarkably successful and has built up a thriving veterinary practice. His achievements so impress the local population that several human patients also request his care. This Orpheus willingly provides, although whether or not his qualifications permit him legally to do so remains unclear.

Orpheus falls in love with, and marries, a gypsy girl, Eurydice (soprano). Eurydice develops a mysterious illness which Orpheus, despite his therapeutic skills, cannot cure. She dies, and is carried away by a cortège of sorrowing animals singing a lament. Three of Eurydice's sisters (mezzo-soprano and two sopranos) then accuse Orpheus of causing her death and stab him. Orpheus dies yearning for his beloved Eurydice.

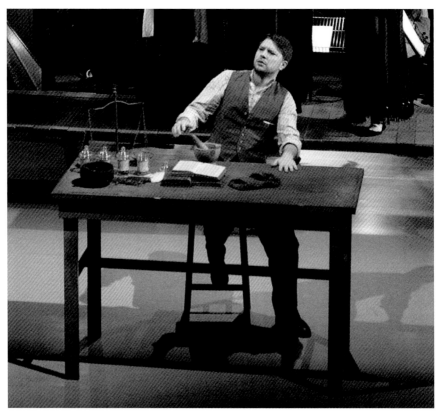

Les Malheurs d'Orphée: Orpheus (Alexey Gusev) in his herbal pharmacy. Royal Conservatoire of Scotland 2017. Photo: Julie Howden.

1. Krohn, R. (ed.), *Gottfried von Strassburg. Tristan – Mittelhochdeutsch, Neuhochdeutsch*, Reclam, Stuttgart, 2007.
2. Weitz, G., 'Love and death in Wagner's *Tristan und Isolde:* an epic anticholinergic crisis', *British Medical Journal* 2003; 327: 1469–71.
3. Robertson, J. I. S., and Weitz, G., *Siegfried's Amnesia: An Attempt at an Explanation*, Scottish Opera, Glasgow, 2015.
4. *The Fish Plaice* in the Saltmarket for those wishing to pursue the matter.
5. A more forthright attempt to assuage sexual desire is made by the evil lapsed knight Klingsor in Wagner's opera *Parsifal*. Klingsor performs on himself bilateral orchidectomy. See p. 36, note 1.
6. Cairns, D. (ed. and trans.), *The Memoirs of Berlioz*, Gollancz, London, 1969, 191–3.

28

MULTIPLE DISEASES AND POLYPHARMACY

A feature of the twenty-first century is increased (and progressively increasing) longevity, with the inevitable concurrent acquisition of multiple ailments calling for treatment with a range of medicines. Together with the mental deterioration and confusion often associated with advancing age, there are frequently created hazards for the patient. This is a situation which has not yet, so far as I am aware, been portrayed in opera. In the following two operas multiple diseases are encountered, but they are fictitious and are proffered by fraudulent imposters.

Haydn's *L'Infedeltà Delusa* of 1773 was composed to a libretto by Marco Coltellini. The spirited young Vespina (soprano) seeks sympathy by disguising herself as a frail old woman and singing of her ailments:

> I've a swelling on my knee
> that forces me to limp,
> An ulcer on the eye
> makes it water all the time.
> I've a cough that's killing me,
> and I can only breathe with pain.

Vespina's supposed maladies are however modestly few in comparison with those allegedly afflicting an elderly lady in Donizetti's *Il Campanello di Notte* (*The Night Bell*) of 1836 composed to his own libretto after the vaudeville *La Sonnette de Nuit* by Brunswick, Troin, and Lhérie (see also pages 52 and 58). It is the wedding night of Don Annibale Pistacchio (bass), a pharmacist. A now disappointed rival, Enrico (baritone), is determined to disrupt consummation of the marriage by making in disguise repeated visits to the pharmacy, ringing the night bell, and demanding urgent prescriptions. In one of these episodes Enrico appears as an elderly gentleman who has come not on his own behalf, but for his wife, who is herself too ill to attend. This is hardly surprising because she is supposedly suffering from diabetes, as a consequence of which she is nearly blind; consumption; intestinal fistulae (seven in number); flatulence; a cerebral tumour; sciatica; and gout. Surprisingly, it does not occur to Don Annibale to question why such an extensive requirement for medicines treating long-standing disorders needs to be made up in the middle of the night. He is, interestingly, rightly concerned not to prescribe mutually incompatible drugs, giving the opera surprisingly vivid contemporary relevance. His work does indeed take several hours, and Don Annibale fails to get back to his bed and his bride. Enrico has won this skirmish.

29

DEMENTIA

As was noted in the last chapter, increased and still increasing longevity is a feature of most Western peoples. Inevitably, this is accompanied by a rising prevalence of dementia, which now affects a substantial proportion of subjects over the age of 65. Early features include memory loss, particularly for recent events, apathy, depression, and diminishing vocabulary. With progression, patients become disorientated, irritable, and ever more dependent on carers. Advanced cases lose speech, cannot recognise even near relatives, are unable to feed themselves, and become incontinent and bedridden.

Some 70 per cent of dementia results from Alzheimer's disease, a condition which features microscopic abnormalities of brain cells and overall shrinkage of the brain. The aetiology is unknown. About 15 to 20 per cent of cases are a consequence of disease of the arteries nourishing the brain. Other causes of dementia are much rarer. Syphilis, once a major reason, is nowadays very unusual (see Chapter 9).

Elena Langer's opera *The Lion's Face* of 2010 is about a patient suffering from dementia, the title referring to the typical leonine facial impassivity of advanced cases. The librettist Glyn Maxwell received substantial guidance from the Institute of Psychiatry at King's College Hospital London, when preparing the text.

The story tells of an elderly man, Mr D (spoken), with severe dementia. He no longer recognises his Wife (mezzo-soprano), whose largely futile attempts at support are aided by a briskly efficient Carer (soprano). A Doctor (baritone) receives from the patient only meaningless answers to questions and is therapeutically ineffective. But the carer's sulky teenage Daughter (soprano), idling because her school is closed for the day, establishes tenuous emotional contact with the patient. Poignantly conveyed is that this is probably the last personal relationship of any kind he will ever have.

Elena Langer's score, irregular and melodically fragmentary, vividly evokes mental chaos. Dramatically most effective is having the patient speak but never sing.

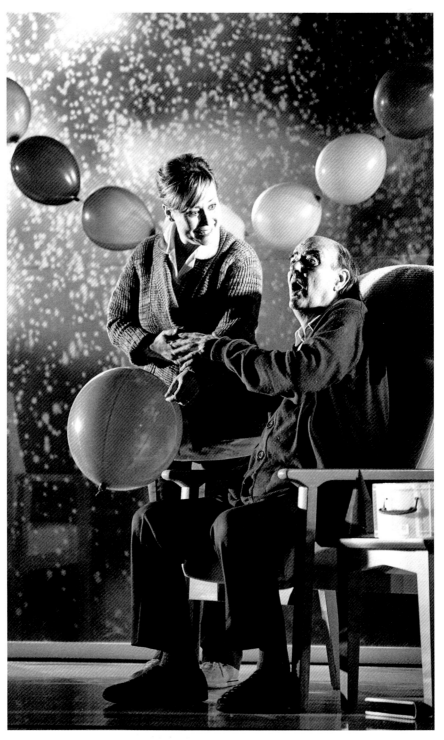

The Lion's Face: The Carer (Rachel Hynes) with the demented patient Mr D (Dave Hill). The Opera Group 2010. Photo: Matthew Andrews.

30

PSYCHIATRIC MUSINGS

Some psychiatric manifestations in opera, such as insanity caused by syphilis and the mass hysteria of the nuns in *The Devils of Loudun*, are diagnostically straightforward. The apparitions seen by the Governess in *The Turn of the Screw* are caused by her temporal lobe epilepsy. In several other operatic situations, aetiology is less clear. Macbeth's vision of the ghost of the murdered Banquo in Act II of Verdi's opera is probably the result simply of a guilty conscience. The derangement of Peter Grimes at the end of that opera is the outcome of horror at the accidental deaths of two of his apprentices.

What became the almost obligatory insertion of a 'mad scene' into operas of the early nineteenth century certainly provided the opportunity for vocal pyrotechnics. It also required the librettist to furnish a plausible cause. The most famous mad scene of all is the soprano Lucia's in Act III of Donizetti's *Lucia di Lammermoor* of 1835. The librettist was Cammarano. Lucia, forcibly married to Arturo (tenor) whom she does not love, has lost her wits and murdered him. Cutting up an unwanted husband into small pieces and then singing about it at great length might seem an extreme reaction, but it allowed Donizetti to compose, and the soprano to sing, some dramatically compelling music.

Effective therapy has in psychiatry lagged behind the advances made in many other medical disciplines. This circumstance is reflected in the psychiatric treatment proffered at various dates depicted in opera. Verdi's *Macbeth* is set in eleventh-century Scotland. The Doctor (bass) advises for the sleepwalking Lady Macbeth (soprano) simply observation and good nursing care. Penderecki's *The Devils of Loudun* has seventeenth-century hysterical nuns supposedly bewitched by various demons. Father Barré (bass) recommends a course of exorcism, to be conducted in public. It would be difficult even to think of an approach less suited to the treatment of hysteria. The nuns' afflictions, predictably, are worsened. Maxwell Davies' *Eight Songs for a Mad King* of 1969 deals with the mental illness of King George III from 1788 to his death in 1820. No firm diagnosis was made then or has been convincingly reached subsequently. The King was treated by a range of doctors who included Sir George Baker, Dr Richard Warren, Sir Lucas

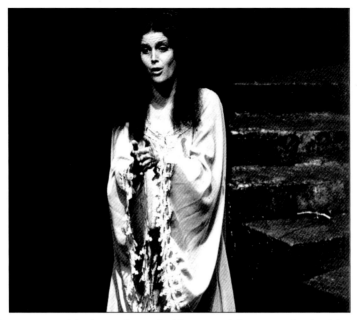

Lucia di Lammermoor: The deranged Lucia (Ashley Putnam), having murdered and dismembered her unwanted husband Arturo, appears before the horrified wedding guests in bloodstained night clothes. Scottish Opera 1981. Photo: Eric Thorburn.

Pepys, Dr Francis Willis and his two sons, and Dr William Heberden the Younger. Therapy, all of which is arbitrary and evidently ineffective, includes forcible restraint, whipping, starvation, harsh purgatives, long walks, and manual labour. Karen MacIver's *The Cabinet of Dr Caligari* of 2016 depicts a Glasgow mental asylum of the late nineteenth century. Treatment comprises mainly brutality and intimidation. Michael Tippett's *The Knot Garden* of 1970 features twentieth-century psychoanalysis and psychotherapy. A more abrasive twentieth century operatic depiction in Murray Schafer's *Requiems for the Party-Girl* of 1972 has Ariadne, a schizophrenic patient in an asylum, surrounded by threatening and incomprehensible figures and eventually killing herself. From the twenty-first century there is Stephen Deazley's *Dream Angus* of 2008, in which psychotherapy is based on the interpretation of dreams; and Philip Venables' *4.48 Psychosis* of 2016, in which depression is treated (ineffectively) with drugs.

It has to be conceded that, in comparison with other disciplines, psychiatric treatment has made very modest advances over the past millennium, although at least frank maltreatment no longer occurs.

Part 3

TWO MORE
OPERATIC DOCTORS

31

A DOCTOR TRAPPED

Thomas Adès's *The Exterminating Angel* is an opera of the absurd, based on the 1962 surreal film of the same title by Luis Buñuel. The libretto is by Tom Cairns in collaboration with Adès.

After an evening at the opera, Edmundo (tenor) and Lucia (soprano) are giving a dinner. Their guests include the star opera singer Leticia (soprano), the conductor Alberto Roc (baritone), the pianist Blanca Delgado (mezzo-soprano), Doctor Carlo Conde (bass-baritone), Señor Russell (baritone), and two engaged lovers, Eduardo (tenor) and Beatriz (soprano). As the guests enter the dining room, several of the servants inexplicably leave. The guests repeat their entrance, further disconcerting the hosts. Dinner is served, albeit much of it is spilled onto the floor. A performing bear and several lambs are removed to the garden. Blanca performs at the piano, delighting the company. When several guests prepare to depart, they become lethargic and distracted. No one attempts to leave and Edmundo graciously offers everyone overnight accommodation. All lie down on the floor to sleep, with Eduardo and Beatriz enthusiastically settling down together in a secluded corner.

The following morning's breakfast is sparse, because no supplies of food have arrived. Dr Conde examines Señor Russell and declares him to be terminally ill. All become increasingly alarmed and fractious when they find themselves inexplicably unable to leave. They are obliged to remain for a second night, during which Russell dies and his corpse is dragged to a closet. Eduardo and Beatriz are noticeably less enthusiastic about their now enforced proximity.

A crowd has by this time gathered outside the house, held back by police, but no one manages to enter. Tormented by thirst, the trapped guests burst open a water pipe. The lambs are retrieved from the garden, slaughtered, cooked on a makeshift fire, and ravenously eaten. Even Dr Conde, thus far the most level-headed, begins to lose his nerve. The bear reappears over the threshold. There are wild suggestions that a human sacrifice is needed. Then Leticia notices that each of the survivors is in exactly the same place as at the start of their mysterious imprisonment. They repeat, so far as they can recall, their actions on that first night. They approach the threshold and cross it to join the crowd outside.

Both orchestration and vocal writing are often bold and scintillating. Adès has set the soprano tessitura demandingly (and abrasively) high, with Leticia at one point being required to sing an A above high C. The première production was enthusiastically praised at the Salzburg Festival, at the Royal Opera House London, and at the Metropolitan Opera New York. Unfortunately, it failed to engage me. Billed as theatre of the absurd, it was indeed absurd and for me devoid of dramatic impact.

32

AN ON-STAGE OPERATIC AUTOPSY

In the second edition of my book *Doctors in Opera: An Irreverent Look at Operatic Medicine*, I discussed the composer Craig Armstrong's opera *The Lady From the Sea*, in which Dr Wangel (tenor) recounts, in unpleasant detail, an autopsy he had previously performed. This was of course described, not enacted. I went on to state that on-stage post-mortem examinations would not provide particularly compelling theatre. In making that assertion I was quite wrong, as shall now be seen.

David Lang's *Anatomy Theater*, to an English libretto by Mark Dion and the composer, was first performed in Los Angeles in June 2017. The events shown are supposed to have taken place in England in the eighteenth century. At that time the bodies of executed criminals were customarily dissected before a paying audience, usually with refreshments served and musicians playing. Organs were removed from the corpse and scrutinized carefully, as it was supposed that anatomical peculiarities could often be detected in criminals, distinguishing them from the normal population. Social superiority of the onlookers was thus emphasized, making the occasion even more jolly. *Anatomy Theater* depicts one such event.

Sarah Osborne (mezzo-soprano) was as a child raped and beaten by her stepfather. Turned out of the house by her mother, she turned to prostitution. She married her pimp, who also then beat her. Sarah murdered the pimp by dosing his drink and smothering him with a pillow. She also killed their two small children. As the opera begins, Sarah stands upon the gallows confessing her crimes. She is then hanged, stripped naked, and publicly dissected. Proceedings are directed medically by Baron Peel (bass-baritone), whose assistant Ambrose Strang (tenor) is required to perform most of the dirty unpleasant duties involved in cutting up a still-warm body. The anatomy theatre's custodian, Jonathan Crouch (baritone), also acts as occasional commentator. Interestingly, Sarah, although ostensibly dead, manages to sing during the procedure. Baron Peel finds that her uterus evinces several marked features denoting criminality.

I was wildly incorrect in suggesting that such activities would not provide vivid theatre. One reviewer considered that *Anatomy Theater*, in a strongly contested field, succeeds in being the goriest of all operas, ever.

Part 4

DOCTORS WRITING ABOUT OPERA

33

DOCTORS WRITING ABOUT OPERA: OPERA VIEWED MEDICALLY

Numerous doctors have written about opera, frequently at length and often, but by no means always, with erudition and discernment. Their contributions have been remarkably diverse.

François Raguenet (c. 1660–1722), born in Rouen, was a doctor and a priest most notable musically for a detailed comparison and critique he published concerning Italian and French music and especially opera of his day, *Paralèle des Italiens et des François, en ce qui regarde la musique et les opéra* (1702). In this, Raguenet strongly favoured the Italians. He praised their instrumentalists' technical training, sight-reading ability, and capability of playing, if necessary, without a conductor. The Italian-born Lully he regarded as the only composer of French opera worthy of note. Raguenet considered Italians to be born musicians, and their castrati indispensable to opera. Hardly surprisingly, Raguenet's observations excited some spirited rejoinders in France. In the resulting polemic, Raguenet was strongly supported by another physician and medical journalist, Nicolas de Boisregard Andry.[1]

William Ashton Ellis (1852–1919) graduated in medicine at St George's Hospital, London. In 1887 he gave up medical practice, and was commissioned by the London Wagner Society to translate into English Wagner's complete prose works. He completed this task in 1899. For many years Ellis's translations were criticized as replicating too closely Wagner's tortured prose construction, with the frequent employment of archaisms and idiosyncratic compound words. Many passages, although ostensibly in English, could seem almost as if still written in a foreign tongue. More recently, Ellis's affinity to the original has come to be seen as more commendable, in capturing an aura of Wagner's writing which a modern translation would lose. Ellis's work remains the standard, and is likely to remain so.[2]

Salvatore Di Giacomo (1860–1934) abandoned medical studies to become a writer. He concentrated on opera and especially on the musical life of Naples from the sixteenth to the eighteenth centuries. His book on the four Neapolitan conservatoires remains a standard reference work. Also published is a collected edition of his articles on opera.[3]

The books on Wagner and Liszt by the Greenock-born composer William Wallace (1860–1940) are discussed on page 16.

The Italian Ulderico Rolandi (1874–1951) was by profession a gynaecologist. He was also a noted music critic and especially a writer on, and collector of, operatic libretti. At his death his accumulation of some 30,000 libretti and 2,000 scores was passed to the Fondazione Giorgio Cini in Venice.[4]

William B. Ober (1920–93) was one of the earliest doctors to take an irreverent view of operatic medicine.[5] He began his article by making the important point that there was neither room nor need for doctors to be included in the cast-lists of classical operas with their gods and goddesses of antiquity, or heroes and heroines of medieval and renaissance legend. Only with Gluck's operatic reforms did the often contrived operatic libretti of the late eighteenth century begin to have characters who could be related to contemporary life.

In the course of his wide-ranging paper, Ober made several perceptive observations. Don Giovanni, in Mozart's opera of that title, has had, if Leporello's catalogue aria is to be believed, sexual exposure to a total of 2,065 women in five countries. Yet he has seemingly and surprisingly escaped venereal infection (AIDS had not appeared in the Don's time). Ober pointed out that many of Wagner's heroines die without apparent cause. As another impious critic put it, in broad Viennese dialect: 'I don't need no dagger; I'll just die on me own.'[6] Death certification would undoubtedly be problematic in a number of Wagner's operas. In Britten's *Death in Venice*, Aschenbach expires quietly sitting in a deckchair on the beach. Although the cause of his death is supposed to be cholera, there is no sign of the profuse watery diarrhoea and dehydration characteristic of the disease. Those features would of course be difficult to portray on stage. Nevertheless, a sudden disturbance of heart rhythm seemed to Ober to be more plausible. In the several operas based on Shakespeare's play *The Merry Wives of Windsor*, Dr Caius is a figure of fun. Yet there lived a real Dr John Caius who very differently was the best-known, and probably the most respected, physician in Tudor England. Ober questioned why Shakespeare decided to denigrate him.

Not all of Ober's observations were correct. He stated that the exact profession of Dr Bartolo in Mozart's *The Marriage of Figaro* and Rossini's *The Barber of Seville* is uncertain. However, the author Beaumarchais makes very clear in the original plays that Bartolo is 'a physician from Seville'.[7]

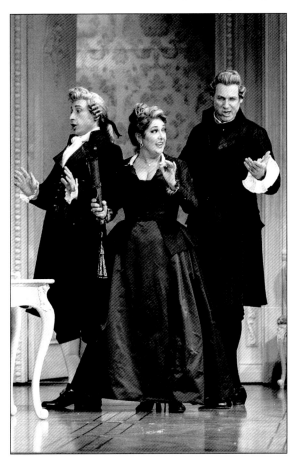

The Marriage of Figaro: Doctor Bartolo (Graeme Broadbent, right) has been summoned to the castle. Expecting to be asked to attend medically on either the Count or the Countess, he finds that he is instead required to provide legal advice to his former mistress Marcellina (Marie McLaughlin). Also present is the music teacher Don Basilio (Paul Curievici). Scottish Opera 2016. Photo: Bill Cooper.

Ober thought that Antonia in *The Tales of Hoffmann* dies from pulmonary tuberculosis. He was of course not alone in believing this. Yet, as I argue in Chapter 18, a cardiac abnormality with disturbance of rhythm is far more likely, as indeed is reflected in the music. These are, however, minor flaws in a penetrating article.

The Russian-born Boris Goldovsky (1908–2001) moved to America in 1930, and between 1946 and 1986 was a prominent opera producer, conductor, impresario, and commentator. He published a very perceptive article on medical aspects of opera.[8] In this he drew particular attention to composers' employment of the orchestra in providing dramatic emphasis in opera. Some specific instances deserve mention. In Mussorgsky's *Boris Godunov* that Tsar's fatal heart attack is made so vivid that nervous members of the audience can involuntarily clutch at their chests (see p. 56). In *Così fan Tutte*, Mozart's use of the woodwinds suggests an almost clinical quivering of the bodies of Ferrando and Guglielmo when Despina applies Dr Mesmer's magnet to draw out their supposed poison. Offenbach's orchestration in *The Tales of Hoffmann* wonderfully conveys Antonia's frenzied excitement as the evil Dr Miracle seizes a violin and incites her and the spectre of her mother to sing. Goldovsky was another of those to consider Antonia's disease to be pulmonary rather than cardiac. When Dr Grenvil takes the pulse of the dying Violetta in the last act of Verdi's *La Traviata*, the audience is informed by the music that her heart rate is 144 beats per minute. The visit of Dr Spinellochio to his supposed patient in Puccini's *Gianni Schicchi* is marked by the contrabassoon executing a coarsely realistic imitation of a bowel movement. I speculated in Chapter 26 on the possible cause of death of Mélisande in Debussy's *Pelléas et Mélisande*. Goldovsky remained uncertain, but accepted that severe bleeding following childbirth, which he perceived as being suggested by her weakness and feeling cold, is not unlikely.

John Carmody[9] took the harsh view that operatic doctors are rarely edifying, although he did concede that Apollo, god of both medicine and music, sets a loftier tone with his appearances in Monteverdi's *Orfeo*, Gluck's *Alceste* and Richard Strauss's *Dafne*. Carmody found the bullying Doctor in Berg's *Wozzeck* and the sinister Dr Miracle in *The Tales of Hoffmann* to be especially repellent. He was critical, as I have also been, of the refusal of Dr Javelinot in Poulenc's *Dialogues des Carmélites* to administer a sufficient dose of drug to relieve the sufferings of the dying Prioress. But Dr Javelinot is fearful of being criticised or disciplined if he risks the life of his patient. He faces a dilemma encountered all too often by doctors treating terminally ill patients today. The law is too harsh; the administration of large doses of pain-relieving medicine should be permitted, even if that hastens the patient's death. Unusually, Carmody considered operatic nurses to be generally more appealing, and sometimes therapeutically more effective, than operatic doctors. The topic of operatic nurses is indeed a delicate one that I have thus far been careful to avoid. He concluded that doctors in opera seem determined to prove the truth of Dr Johnson's aphorism that opera is an exotic and irrational entertainment.

Erik St Louis, then a third-year medical student, made a comparison of three divergent twentieth-century operatic doctor–patient relationships.[10] He took Berg's *Wozzeck*, in which the bullying Doctor employs the impoverished Wozzeck as a subject for his hare-brained dietary research; Debussy's unfinished *La Chute de la Maison Usher*, in which the Doctor, evincing a mixture of perplexity and low cunning, mistakes one of Madeline's cataleptic trances for her death; and Michael Nyman's *The Man Who Mistook His Wife for a Hat*, which has the kindly, perceptive Dr S correctly diagnosing visual agnosia, a rare abnormality in which the patient is able to see, but unable to recognize or identify, what is seen. In the opinion of St Louis, only in the third opera is a proper relationship developed and established between patient and doctor. As St Louis concluded, 'Dr S demonstrates a flexible, compassionate attitude, which better enables fiduciary duties towards his patient ... to be met.'

J. Worth Estes, in an exposition notable for its scholarship and detailed documentation,[11] examined the changing role of operatic doctors over the years. He found that all of the uncomplimentary portrayals of physicians are in operas whose plots date from before about 1830. After that, increasingly favourable views of the medical profession begin to appear in the wake of the first major advances in the therapeutic capability of doctors. He concluded that physicians (and presumably surgeons) on the operatic stage are best understood as reflections of how the authors of the dramas being acted out there perceived the medical profession of their own times.

Michael Hutcheon, a professor of medicine at the University of Toronto, together with his wife Linda Hutcheon, a professor of English, in 1996 published their book *Opera: Desire, Disease, Death*. This work, together with some reviews it received in the medical literature, is discussed on page 1.

Michael O'Donnell[12] came closest to the irreverent approach I adopted in my book on operatic doctors, speaking of 'those minor characters ... whose on-stage professional performance would be quite unacceptable off it ... opera ... offers wholly unacceptable role models'. I agree with O'Donnell that many, if not most, operatic doctors are disreputable. But there are some worthy, and hence noteworthy, exceptions.

The review by Stephen Lock[13] was broader, and less concerned with doctors as operatic characters than with the diseases occurring in opera. This was to be expected in an article in a medical textbook. Thus, tuberculosis, syphilis, cholera, and plague are prominent. At the date of his writing, no opera about HIV/AIDS had appeared, but Lock predicted that one would soon arrive. He was right; Eötvös's *Angels in America* had its première performance in 2004.

Stefan Willich[14] reverted broadly to the approach made earlier by Estes, examining physicians in operas over the years as a reflection of medical history and public perception. Willich showed again that in the eighteenth century operatic physicians do not have a healing function but often play the buffoon in a socially subordinate and purely supportive role. In the early nineteenth century there appears the miracle doctor and charlatan. Later nineteenth-century doctors are often presented as scientifically trained, albeit that rise in competence and power has the potential to be employed detrimentally. In the twentieth century the doctor can have a major role. As well as clinician, he may undertake research.

Usually he now possesses higher social status. Willich made no comment concerning operatic doctors of the twenty-first century.

Two articles by Gunther Weitz, concerning the administration of potions containing extracts of plants of the solanaceae (belladonna) family in the operas *Tristan und Isolde* and *Götterdämmerung*, are discussed in Chapter 27.

Finally, there is of course the present author.

1. Cohen, A., and Sadie, J. A., *Grove* III, 1216.
2. Cormack, D., in Vazsonyi, N. (ed.), *The Cambridge Wagner Encyclopedia*, Cambridge University Press, Cambridge, 2013, 112–13.
3. Tammaro, F., *Grove* I, 1175–6.
4. *Grove* IV, 11–12.
5. Ober, W. B., 'Operatic "doctors"', *The Practitioner* 1976; 216: 110–16.
6. Nestroy, J. Quoted by Gál, H. in *Richard Wagner*, Stein & Day, New York, 1976, 154.
7. Beaumarchais, P., *The Barber of Seville* and *The Marriage of Figaro*. Translated by Wood, J., Penguin Books, London, 1964.
8. Goldovsky, B., 'Some Medical Matters in Operatic Literature', *Cleveland Clinic Quarterly* 1986; 53: 39–43.
9. Carmody, J., 'Doctors and Opera', *The Medical Journal of Australia* 1991; 155: 783–4.
10. St Louis, E. K., 'The Physician in Contemporary Opera: Three Divergent Approaches to the Doctor–Patient Relationship', *The Pharos* 1992; 55: 15–20.
11. Estes, J. W., 'The Changing Role of the Physician in Opera', *Opera Quarterly* 1994; 10: 143–55.
12. O'Donnell, M., 'On Not Giving a Figaro', *Health and Ageing*, November 2000, 48.
13. Lock, S., 'Opera', in *The Oxford Illustrated Companion to Medicine*, edited by Lock, S., Last, J. M., and Dunea, G., Oxford University Press, Oxford, 2001, 593–4.
14. Willich, S. N., 'Physicians in Opera: Reflection of Medical History and Public Perception', *British Medical Journal* 2006: 333: 1333–5.

INDEX